know
it is but i
don't think
it's **serious**

Confidence and
decisiveness
in primary care

I don't know what it is but I don't think it's **serious**

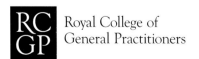

Royal College of
General Practitioners

Tim Crossley

The Royal College of General Practitioners was founded in 1952 with this object:
'To encourage, foster and maintain the highest possible standards in general practice and for that purpose to take or join with others in taking steps consistent with the charitable nature of that object which may assist towards the same.'

Among its responsibilities under its Royal Charter the College is entitled to:
'Diffuse information on all matters affecting general practice and issue such publications as may assist the object of the College.'

British Library Cataloguing-in-Publication Data
A catalogue record for this book is available from the British Library

© Royal College of General Practitioners 2008
Published by the Royal College of General Practitioners 2008
14 Princes Gate, Hyde Park, London SW7 1PU

Disclaimer
This publication is intended for the use of medical practitioners in the UK and not for patients. The authors, editors and publisher have taken care to ensure that the information contained in this book is correct to the best of their knowledge, at the time of publication. Whilst efforts have been made to ensure the accuracy of the information presented, particularly that related to the prescription of drugs, the authors, editors and publisher cannot accept liability for information that is subsequently shown to be wrong. Readers are advised to check that the information, especially that related to drug usage, complies with information contained in the *British National Formulary*, or equivalent, or manufacturers' datasheets, and that it complies with the latest legislation and standards of practice.

Designed and typeset by Robert Updegraff
Printed by Latimer Trend
Indexed by Carol Ball

ISBN: 978-0-85084-318-7

Contents

Preface

Decisiveness

Around 1992 huge computers first started appearing on GPs' desks, largely it seemed to make our prescriptions more legible. We had not started to use them for record keeping or data entry of any kind.

Not long after the 'monster' had landed on my desk, a man whom I'd seen recently consulted me, looking very pleased.

'That computer', he launched off, 'is bloody brilliant.'
'Really?' I was not sure where this was going.
'Yeah, the tablets it chose for me were absolutely fantastic....'

Medical decision making is sometimes taken to mean coming to an important, strategic-level conclusion and agreed action on a big issue, with long-term results. It contrasts with problem solving, which is smaller in scale, deals with personal, individual matters for which there might be a single correct answer (if only one was good enough at it) and has immediate consequences. But we live with uncertainty, as the cliché has it, and we acknowledge therefore that we are unable to Solve Problems at times, and Decisions are even tougher. It is inescapable.

GPs, despite the increasingly structured consultations driven by the Quality and Outcomes Framework (QOF), and despite the progress made with developing a clear curriculum, have to handle this uncertainty. Indeed the curriculum specifies this as a skill in itself (Domain 3). On the other hand the perception is that we live in a society less able to handle uncertainty, or 'fate', and simultaneously less certain of what a GP is actually capable of doing to relieve this.

We have always had some doctors who are more confident than others, merely as a reflection of the spectrum of humanity. The aim of this book is to be both broadly analytical of the underlying issues (from our own, society's and the patients' view) and practical in looking at the points in our work where uncertainty can be managed better. This includes both within the consultation (especially in the appropriate reassurance phase) and in our non-clinical responsibilities where the indecisive, uncertain doctor also struggles.

Medical decision making is difficult, and to be confident despite uncertainties even more so. This book challenges doctors in primary care, who are at the forefront of medical care, whether in training or established in practice, to understand and deal with the uncertainties they see every day.

The book is lightly referenced and I hope lightly written, with anecdotes and personal accounts of situations any practising GP will recognise. This is real life.

Tim Crossley FRCGP
July 2008

Foreword 1

I first read the draft of this book midway through my registrar days and then later as an independent, 'fresh' GP. The book should appeal particularly to GP registrars and those of us starting out in practice. However, more experienced GPs will also recognise Tim's themes of medical decisiveness and clarity, even those who view all those changes in our health system with mixed feelings – confusion of role, sadness, bewilderment, shock, and maybe a bit of cynicism about guidelines and protocols.

The problem is not with those guidelines but with the majority of our patients who seem to take a perverse pleasure in not following them. Perhaps this reflects our medical training, still focused on the biological model of illness without fully encompassing the psycho-social model. Tim emphasises this in his characteristic style – humorous, philosophical and without mincing words. He uses many anecdotes, some amusing and others sad, to serve as learning points.

The wide variety of unusual cases (such as the man who eats newspapers) as well as the wide range of common cases, complicated by issues like unrealistic expectations and the psycho-social make-up of the patient, make our speciality quite different from hospital medicine, and with particular challenges. To identify the 'real problem' of the patient from the mild organic pathology that he or she has presented is daunting yet exciting, like your first few attempts at solving Rubik's cube. You can quickly make a little progress but then get stuck. How do GPs make progress beyond this? This sense of how to make confident decisions – even why the patient has chosen us, of all people, to help them do that – is the core of the book.

The later chapters cover issues like complaints, difficult colleagues and personal organisation. This is most enlightening for registrars, even though they have 'management' training elsewhere. Many of the observations and comments stem from his own experiences as an enthusiast and educationalist. Knowing Tim as someone who is usually brutally honest and straightforward, but also cleverly subtle at times, I have this tip to offer for the readers: read the book once and then again as there is more to be learnt and enjoyed by 'reading between the lines'.

Dr Asha Thomas MRCGP
July 2008

Foreword 2

Being a general practitioner is a highly satisfying and privileged job that allows us to interact with many people in many different ways. The diversity and scope of family medicine means that no two days are ever the same. Whilst this is enormously intellectually and emotionally stimulating, the realisation that as a GP you really do need to know 'a little bit about everything' is a daunting prospect even for the most self-assured.

It goes without saying that patients should have confidence in their GP, but less talked about and equally as important is that GPs have confidence in themselves. The ever-changing NHS, the sheer breadth of clinical knowledge we need to keep abreast of and the shifting dynamic of the doctor–patient relationship combine to make this increasingly difficult.

But perhaps the worst – and all too frequent – challenge we GPs face is that of having to make decisions in the absence of certainty. While experience forces us to accept that uncertainty is a fact of life, this book offers a glimmer of light at the end of the tunnel. Using anecdotes and examples from real life, it provides practical advice on areas of our work where uncertainty and ambiguity can be managed better, both inside and outside the consulting room.

Crucially, the book recognises that being confident in medical decision making doesn't mean blindly flailing towards a diagnosis. Rather, by weighing up the evidence, working in partnership with the patient and sharing our anxieties with colleagues we can act decisively, safe in the knowledge that the patient's trust in our judgement is well-founded.

Professor Steve Field
Chair of Council, Royal College of General Practitioners
July 2008

Acknowledgements

This book has materialised out of working with many fantastic people. I have had the pleasure of teaching about 20 GP registrars, all of whom have been influential. My partners, past and present, continue to educate me.

I am particularly and specifically grateful to Alison Watson, Dominic Faux and Asha Thomas, who all read the book and gave helpful feedback including on style and grammar.

The book has been carefully read (and re-read), and edited, by Rodger Charlton, who with colleagues at the College has turned the book from an interesting idea into I hope something useful and effective. I am enormously grateful for this support.

But my wife, Dami, also a GP trainer and in the same inner-city practice as me, has been fabulous and endlessly supportive. She has spent many hours listening and coping and advising.

To her, this book is proudly dedicated.

Abbreviations

A&E	accident and emergency
ALL	acute lymphoblastic leukaemia
AML	acute myeloid leukaemia
BMA	British Medical Association
BNP	beta-type natriuretic peptide
BP	blood pressure
BSE	bovine spongiform encephalopathy
CJD	Creutzfeldt–Jakob disease
COPD	chronic obstructive pulmonary disease
CPD	Continuing Personal Development
CPN	community psychiatric nurse
CT	computed tomography
DENS	doctor's educational needs
DVT	deep-vein thrombosis
EBM	evidence-based medicine
ECG	electrocardiogram
ECT	electroconvulsive therapy
ENT	ear, nose and throat
GMC	General Medical Council
HA	health authority
HMO	health maintenance organisation
IBS	irritable bowel syndrome
ITU	intensive therapy unit
LMC	Local Medical Committee
MCQs	multiple-choice questions
MDT	multi-disciplinary team
MI	myocardial infarction
MMR	measles, mumps and rubella
NICE	National Institute for Health and Clinical Excellence
NSAID	non-steroidal anti-inflammatory drug
PBC	Practice-Based Commissioning
PCO	Primary Care Organisation
PDP	Personal Development Plan
PE	pulmonary embolus
PEC	Professional Executive Committee
PHCT	primary healthcare team
PPI	proton pump inhibitor
PSA	prostate specific antigen
PUNS	patient's unmet needs
RAM	Rapid Access Memory
RTA	road traffic accident
SHO	senior house officer
STD	sexually transmitted disease
URTI	upper respiratory tract infection

CHAPTER 1

Confident decision making

GPs are expected to draw sensible, authoritative conclusions from a mix of confounding, unusual and also mundane information, and to develop those conclusions with confidence and decisiveness. Registrars and experienced doctors are equally bemused by the challenges of decision making in the absence of certainty.

Confidence and decisiveness are similar ideas, and we perhaps look at these in other professions with envy. This chapter introduces the ideas of medical self-confidence, the need to share in decisions, and the necessity of sound communication skills in achieving that.

I had a patient who liked to eat newspapers. He came to the surgery, perfectly fit and well, and said he enjoyed the taste of newsprint and liked to swallow small pieces. Was this a problem? He'd only come because his wife was alarmed at the lifelong habit. He was well, and in other ways had an average, unremarkable office job and lifestyle.

Primary care is full of this stuff. The pleasure of the job is in large measure the variety and weirdness of the presentations and the knowledge that, no matter who writes the hottest new computer program, the best coding system and the fastest NHS Direct protocol, nothing will prepare us for some patients – perhaps quite a high proportion of them. We are not indispensable but we are wired better than anyone else for the unexpected. It tests us and, though I am using this possibly trivial case, our capacity for finding a sensible way forward is a particular feature of general practice.

Obviously, in this instance, one wants to do everything one can for the patient, and take a good history. (It is hard to suppress the temptation to indulge in a bit of flippancy, asking if the quality papers taste better. And what about the Sunday supplements? Are some articles more digestible than others? But we manage.)

In the absence of physical problems we move on to what, exactly, was on his and his wife's mind? Does he have any other odd habits? Information is limited; he is not very articulate. Common sense suggests that the paper is unlikely to be harmful in small amounts, but the ink is more complex. We are talking milligram quantities however. A phone call to the poisons centre proves reassuring, and, straight faced, we can pass on the judgement that the accidental consumption of much larger amounts of ink are thought to be OK though the evidence is sparse.

So we are back to a GP judgement. Do we tell him it is fine? Do we say, as obviously many relatives have, that it is silly and might possibly be dangerous? Is it our job to dish out common sense and wisdom? Experience suggests we might not be getting the whole truth and we don't want to misjudge the problem by implicitly condoning all sorts of other odd eating habits. Are we witnessing the start of a mental health problem? In fact is the patient, the person with a medical need, the one in front of us or the anxious wife?

Twenty minutes have gone by. We fudge it, knowing that our safety net is in place, and move on to more solid ground: a patient with hypertension.

Observer bias and real-life patients

If you believe something is going to happen then it makes it more likely to occur. This is why sensible research separates the one doing the measuring from the scientist who remains 'blind' because the results are biased by the scientist's belief. I have always thought this sounded almost corrupt but the rigging of the figures is of course an unconscious process, and we are all prone to it.

Think about this the next time you check a blood pressure (BP) in a nervous patient who is on treatment for hypertension. You have an old-fashioned mercury sphygmomanometer.

First, you have a relationship with the patient even if this is a new encounter. The youngest medical and nursing graduates might find themselves excited by an interesting case of whatever, but those who survive any time in the health service soon prefer to see well people rather than ill ones, and are saddened by disease rather than thrilled by it.

So you don't want to find a high BP with connotations of imminent (or at any rate premature) vascular catastrophe. You are with the patient on this one. Then as the mercury drops, rather more hastily than the recommended 2 mm per second, you listen for the first Korotkoff sound and you have to decide if it was the very first little puff of pulse detected or was it the firmer thud heard 10 mm lower down? You glance at the previous record and see the result last time was a few mm lower still; which do you record today? The last recording was by you, presumably in the same haste, so could have been uncertain; however, noting a duplicate of the lower result makes it appear rock-solid definite. This is a serious moment and, with the modern belief in obsessive poly-pharmaceutical control, the implications are considerable. A lower result might mean not adding a third or fourth drug (side effects, cost, hassle) or deciding on deferred elective surgery, or more Quality and Outcomes Framework (QOF) points of the new 2004 GP contract. It might be better to use the automatic electronic meter – but that gives the higher result, which you didn't want. Was the cuff microphone correctly positioned and the cuff the right size? Oh dear. Perhaps just check it again next time.

Time-consuming interval measurements and intensive efforts at therapy are seen as Best Practice. Yet not only do they seem impractical in real life but also one is easily convinced that creating less palaver is in the patient's and the population's interest.

Is this colluding with the patient's denial? No; because we know this is not perfect and the result we record today is merely an estimate. We know our observations are of limited value and that many other factors are at play in the effort to keep the patient healthy. The sensible GP weighs up these issues and discusses the findings; the unconfident doctor focuses on the number and chews at it and it alone.

Well, we want to be a confident GP so what are our findings and options?

- We might confidently tell the patient that his or her blood pressure is no problem and leave it at that. This is taking the whole responsibility on our own shoulders. Usually it works. It is arguably stretching the truth, but at the margins of target blood pressure the numbers needed to treat are at least 100 – i.e. if we say the patient's BP at 151/96 is satisfactory and not going to harm him or her in the next decade we will be right over 99 per cent of the time.

- We might choose to tell the patient that there *is* a problem and we must re-check to see what is to be done. There is the option to pass this re-check on to either a practice nurse who will respect the protocols much more than we do, or the keen new partner who is better informed on the latest thinking and remains unburdened by an excess of experience. This option of course crosses one's mind but is suitably dismissed.

- Or perhaps we should muddle along after all, for isn't this the truth of 'masterly inactivity', not being entirely clear with our nervous patient and not letting him or her catch our eye when we start to pack the machine up. We console ourselves that we have not lied; we would tell the truth if we were asked. But because we might become paternalistic communicators, and know how to avoid the patient's eye, we are not faced with a clear request for the truth, and even if we are we don't share the whole truth. Not in the sense meant in a court.

- Another option would be about sharing our anxieties with the patient. Expressing perhaps not only anxiety for the patient's health but also for the therapeutic dilemma you are trying not to face.

- We could defer it all. One of the pleasures of primary care is the paucity of true crashing emergencies: we nearly always have time to assemble more information, such as going and looking things up in a book, a website or a guideline. An alternative route to further information comes by a referral, as certainly any hospital physician would manage this patient via a number of hospital-type tests on a rather more intensive basis than the way we do it. For sure they would increase the treatment given to the patient. And somehow the evidence-based medicine information does not seem to apply in this particular case on this particular morning.

Much of the direction of this decision will be led by GPs' characteristics. Are they risk-averse, driven by QOF points, keen on population management-type doctors? Are they sceptics of the value of the last little drop in blood pressure when the white-coat effect seems pretty evident, the numbers needed to treat to avert one event in a population with a blood pressure just above the threshold for treatment is well into three figures, and the particular patient in front has already tried several antihypertensives and has had problems with them already? Has the GP had problems with his or her own blood pressure? And what is his or her philosophical position on the extent to which decisions can be passed on to patients?

If a decision as clear cut as the management of simple hypertension is capable of tying us in knots, then how do we tackle the completely bewildering presentation in primary care? And yet we would hate the job if it failed to produce variety, so somehow we develop tools to make a start on almost anything.

4   A confident society

Confident decision making starts with an understanding of what confidence is.

Western capitalist society is built on confidence on a huge and grand scale. The wealth of the West is built on the trust that things get better. Stocks go up, and people feel able to risk borrowing more to spend on goods. That makes someone else richer, so our net collective value goes up. So stocks go up more. Feeling good about paper wealth generates more paper wealth, so when the housing market is rising at all, it tends to rise sharply.

It is a convenient human failing to discard evidence that conflicts with a general level of optimism which normally sustains us – until some inescapable event, tragedy or report hints at a more difficult future that then puts the system into reverse for a while. Tom Wolfe in his excellent novel *The Bonfire of the Vanities* details the seeping, then surging loss of confidence colleagues had in his anti-hero, the financier Sherman McCoy.[1] That the decline was due to essentially unrelated, irrelevant problems shows the irrationality of the system. But the costs both financial and personal, as his city deals unravelled through a vicious circle of lack of faith, lost confidence and reduced performance, were enormous.

An awful lot of very clever and well-informed people drive the price of stocks, yet despite much effort they cannot accurately judge risk in their financial planning. So the day-to-day value of stocks is largely judged by confidence and rumour, which is about as far as you can get from rationality. Yet it works, sort of, with reservations. And it is fun having an unpredictable future. We accept that alongside those advertisements for a sports car (promising all sorts of performance, including a reverse gear under the driver's control) is another for a tax-efficient investment scheme (promising some, hoping for plenty, yet pointing out in the small printout that the uncontrolled reverse gear can be a problem).

Crime is a problem second only to the social consequences of fear of crime. The most likely victims of violence (young black male) do not fit the tabloid image (old pathetic female).[2] Rationalising risk is very difficult though – women doctors feel more threatened than men but they are not in reality at higher risk, and might be lower as they are less likely to be confrontational. Behaviour such as avoiding home visits or night work through this fear is difficult to alter.

Teachers rule through having the confidence to be assertive. There seems in the confident teacher an ability to command respect such that the pupil, whether he or she admits it or not, wishes to please him. But there is also an atmosphere, a tension, in which there is an unspoken and possibly ill-defined threat of an undesirable consequence to disrespect. This is not violence of the sort favoured in the more medieval public schools, but a sanction of some sort – and what is more fearsome than the unknown? – available to the confident teacher. The teacher's skill in crowd control, if not as an educator, is in manipulating this atmosphere, giving an impression that calling his or her bluff is not a wise option. And then turning the mob's attention to the issue in hand, learning, without having meted out any punishment at all.

> I had a maths teacher whose certainty in his subject and in the methods he used to teach were awesome. We were all frightened of him, though he was never violent and did not raise his voice. He was physically fit, spending lunch-breaks sweating around the running track, startling the smoking clique. His lessons were very controlled and precise, with a clear outcome and very clear boundaries.
>
> Maths might be the only true certainty and it might be an interesting study to compare, say, tolerance of uncertainty in maths teachers with perhaps their colleagues in the economics department.
>
> His nickname was Killer. I know of no evidence that he actually killed anyone but neither I nor anyone else had any desire to test him.

Every GP has a nervous teacher patient whose confidence has cracked open in the cruel classroom. There seems a special empathy with these unappreciated public servants, whose authority has proven to be ephemeral.

The problem for clinicians is that people want to know the future and alter it in their favour with some confidence; we know that this can only be done on a population basis (the country is generally getting healthier), not an individual one (stocks can go down as well as up). But if the clinician expresses too much uncertainty he or she feels unworthy and nervous, and patients pick this up.

The failure of clinical confidence

The number of doctors (and nurses) not working at any one time is terrifying.[3] The catch-all reason for early retirements and part-time working without children to blame is 'morale' or 'stress'.

Is it fair to say that many clinicians avoid clinical decision making or work itself through lack of confidence? Clearly our psychological morbidity is high.[4] But are we mixing the sense of stress and pressure with formal diagnoses of mental illness (whether work related or not)?

> You might not feel it, but compared with your patients you are well-off financially. And the retail trade knows it, which is why a salesperson who learns how you earn a crust will feel a twinge of chest tightening as the sweet odour of a commission flares his nostrils and brightens his eyes.
>
> You are bright, brighter in fact, than the salesperson, but this does not deter his or her confident patter. He or she has reason to be confident,

after all, because there is something you want even if you don't know it yet, and the salesperson knows that he or she might be able to supply it. He or she has self-belief and you rather admire it.

Salespeople use a myriad of techniques but consider the ones who have sold you things that turn out to be not quite what you expected in quality and usefulness: the clothes worn but once, or the car that loses excitement within a thousand miles. And the kitchen gadget – a variation of the spinning blade on a motor-type – with a highly restricted and specialised use. Their utter pointlessness baffles you when you get home. Do you blame the salespeople? Are you cross with them? Or does a little bit of you rather admire them?

Sales of such goods are not made by using high-pressure forces such as those employed by the notorious door-to-door double-glazing and encyclopaedia companies. The sales staff who are effective with you are likely to be well-informed and helpful, working in their own attractive surroundings. Good staff are carefully honest with their claims and manage to give the feeling that you are on the same side, that they understand you and can help, and they acknowledge that not everything in the shop or showroom is right for you – getting this idea across engenders more confidence in you because you feel that they are not uncritical, that they can hold an objective viewpoint. So you like them, and sufficient trust develops to allow the sale to be clinched.

The marketing of private health care is part of the same pattern. The private sector has one undeniable advantage – speed or convenience of delivery (often the same thing) – but the patients might believe they are getting a better product. There is no evidence that an operation is any better or safer at a private hospital, but many patients believe it to be so. To be fair to the sector such claims are not made, indeed denied, but all primary care staff, who do the referring, know the patients' motivations are complex. The atmosphere of barely subdued opulence and calm control makes the private reception and ward staff's job easier. The operation goes better because the patient is more contented. On another occasion the sale of, say, complete check-ups for asymptomatic healthy middle-aged people is smoothed. This is despite the lack of evidence of effectiveness of such procedures. Indeed, in my experience, the excitement of being told you are well wears off in well under a thousand miles.

General Household Survey questionnaires on GPs demonstrate a correlation between job satisfaction and high scores, but the researchers are careful to say that, whilst GPs like junior doctors are scoring 2–3, which apparently suggests 50 per cent have a definable psychiatric condition, this cannot be conclusive without secondary psychiatric interviews. The general population figures are 20–30 per cent psychiatric morbidity (which itself has massive implications for philosophers, novelists and others who strive to define human normality). In other words doctors are unhappy, and readily admit to symptoms on a questionnaire validated with the general population. But we cannot deduce that they are more ill in much larger numbers than the general population.[5,6]

The numbers retiring hurt from medicine are hard to ascertain, not least because of the political charge attached to them. After spending hundreds of thousands of pounds on training, it is rather too painful for the Department of Health to confess its failure rate in public. The British Medical Association (BMA) is happy to generate figures in its annual information to the Review Boards but we have to be sceptical.

More anecdotally still is the resistance to change seen by varying degrees in doctors.[7]

This is exemplified by the way appointment systems work as discussed in the later chapter on coping with politicians and managers. Essentially, doctors tend to want to keep control of the system, and, except in a small organisation like a well-defined single-handed practice, fail. This is unhelpful for their confidence and makes Mondays even worse than they are already.

Money obviously is an issue too in that, if the opportunity to have a reasonable standard of living is there regardless of workload, the temptation is strong. And many doctors marry other doctors, or professionals with a decent income.

So let us not blame morale and stress for everything. A large cohort of trained clinicians have a life outside the consulting room and, whilst not necessarily avoiding clinical work because it is too stressful, nevertheless are not tempted to work (or work more) because the core of their duties is not enjoyable. There is a difference.

The thousands of extra doctors and nurses in the current NHS Plan are not going to appear from universities this side of the next government by the nature (i.e. length) of their training. The European Union countries and other sources of oven-ready clinicians are of value, but linguistic and cultural barriers are not diminishing. Efforts clearly have to be made to get the locally trained clinicians to work to avoid perpetuating all those NHS delivery problems.

That, of course, is someone else's problem and no service will run well on a mixture of guilt and a Protestant work ethic alone, but I hope to kindle some idealism and self-belief in individual doctors. Here there is a concordance between the needs of the NHS and of the clinician.

Humiliation of students

'And finally, Mr Crossley, finally; that tie does not go with that shirt. Did your mother not tell you that?'

This was from an orthopaedic surgeon, now a professor, who epitomised the kind of arrogant bedside teaching that was prevalent when I was a student in the 1970s. It continues today, though I believe less commonly.

The perpetrators of this kind of approach are often accomplished and clever clinicians, good doctors and nurses, whatever that means. But they are almost wholly untrained teachers and poor observers of humanity.

The medical model of bedside teaching by humiliation has a number of aims. As well as the simple pleasure of crushing a student, it is to demonstrate superior knowledge in the teacher and therefore respect. It is important in an animal way to re-assert the pecking order within the tribe. The teacher is aiming for the role of, as it were, the senior breeding male. These aims are best achieved with a large formal setting, where the audience consists of staff of all ranks hovering around. The 'teacher' then picks on a student and asks questions until they can't answer any more. This is quite easy to do, in that questioners can easily think of a fact or item of knowledge they possess, ask the student for it and if he or she answers correctly go for the next fact laying beneath it. A request for an explanation of a symptom, for instance, is then answered with a list of possibilities from which questioners select one, asking for causes, strategies, numbers, references or whatever. You can look quite knowledgeable if you keep the upper hand in the game.

Meanwhile the student's aim is to avoid eye contact, and if caught try to survive the questions somehow. But of course there is an inevitability of getting to the one that cannot be answered. So long as the sequence has got to a reasonably obscure depth, if not the very bottom, rather like in pot-holing, then some honour might be retained.

I was never a good student, and orthopaedics was pretty low on my undistinguished list of interests and successes at the time.

But there are two thoughts that emerge from the truly terrible memory of that ward round at which I was flattened. The first is that I recall the subject matter was the meaning and value of temperature charts at the end of the bed in a postoperative patient. I knew too little and the barking surgeon, having demonstrated my ignorance, undeniably showed me a gap in useful knowledge that I later filled. For years as a houseman I thought of him when looking over a temperature chart. Not infrequently I found I was better at interpreting them than colleagues. So I have reluctantly to admit that some learning took place.

The second point is that I fancy myself to be fairly robust mentally (or at least have no insight into my psychopathology) and this ridicule as well as other lesser episodes did not put me off medicine or patients, merely the medical hierarchy. Some students of a more sensitive disposition bear deeper scars in their working lives. So why do clever people like this man do it? One wonders if like the playground bully such 'teachers' are themselves victims, themselves unconfident in who and what they are. Why else round off such a diatribe with personal abuse?

What do patients want?

Others must discuss the overlap between what is wanted and what is needed. However, the room for conflict is vast and so an understanding of a patient's wants is vital to any successful clinical interaction, even if that set of wants is not what is actually provided or what the doctor would describe as needed. The more sophisticated phrase to describe these is 'ideas, concerns and expectations' and GPs need a profound understanding of this area. The patient has his or her set of these and perhaps some goals, but will often choose to voice them very indirectly. The doctor has his or her thoughts, of course, but experience shows how just saying them bluntly is rarely the most successful tactic. Really there is a diplomatic chess game going on here.

The art of diplomacy is to get the other side to suggest, as if it was their idea in the first place, what you wanted in the first place. The game rules state clearly that the other side should not know or be directly told what your desired outcome is, certainly in the first round. Diplomacy is also about making a judgement when to concede that the other side is going to do what they are going to do anyway and trying to have some respect for it.

Primary care particularly requires intense diplomatic skills. Doctors also need to know when to avoid the game, and allow the patient to trust them.

In an individual case the art of getting reluctant patients to take their treatments is to get *them* to suggest they need them. In order to do this each patient has to be encouraged to feel safe in letting the GP know his or her agenda, without being embarrassed or feeling it is some kind of test. The jargon term in GP communication studies and work is 'eliciting health beliefs' and it is difficult for both the patient and the person taking the history. But time and again the reward for asking a patient his or her health beliefs, in a safe atmosphere, is a surprising response. He or she might be three steps ahead of you or have gone down a completely different track.

The one thing that seems too much to ask for in patients is cold rationality. After all, the pleasure of smoking cannot be rationally said to outweigh the consequences in terms of money never mind health, yet a quarter of adults still do it. And when, in communicating with our patients, we find that suddenly they flip from wanting to be the leader in choosing the next step to demanding certainty and dogma from us, we should at least understand it. Whilst it seems at least partially like sidestepping the responsibility to keep pushing them to decide, it is really sharing the load.

A fine example of the kind of irrational approach to health choices in public health is the treatment of serious mental health problems in the community. The absolute volume of evidence in favour is immense and the sheer experience with it is great. But politicians who contemplate promoting this for their area and closing hospital beds are afraid of the journalist who asks for a guarantee that no one will come to any harm. So they ask the managers and mental health people to promise that all will go well because it feels rather risky to them, and the reply is that it will, that patients do much better when helped in the community, that reports of harm to anyone else in the community are much exaggerated....

But guarantees are difficult.

(Interestingly there is a valid argument to be had about autonomy and compulsory treatment of a population in the community, and about keeping the hospital options available. But the scientific evidence is overwhelmingly on one side: good community care works well. Then again the scientific evidence for banning cigarettes is vast. Since this book has been written, a ban on smoking in all workplaces in England and Wales has been implemented, showing an encouraging respect for the facts by the politicians.)

Now guarantees when issued by, say, Vauxhall, are not a promise that the car will work beautifully for whatever period. They are a promise that they will put right a problem at no cost and minimal hassle, and they can make it because they know most of their cars will in fact be fine. The average cost of repairs done under guarantee is known with some accuracy and therefore the occasional costly repair is met perfectly happily (for them if not the customer). Medicine of course cannot put right every consequence so we either have to promise nothing will go wrong – or not issue guarantees in the consumer sense of the term.

Our public health doctor if he was more confident might be able to say, given the colossal weight of evidence in favour of community care, that previous experience has been that in a population hundreds of times bigger than the one contemplating the change, over some years, no reported harm has resulted. The number of people struck by lightning on the other hand is much larger. The confident doctor can inject some rationality into the decision without belittling the population and their representatives' lack of statistical nous. It is a fine art because to put across confidence in the science, as discussed later in the book, without being dogmatic, legalistic, a pedant or fluffing it all up with jargon is very difficult.

Is confidence necessarily desirable?

Too much confidence is arrogance and a failure to reflect on ourselves critically is a clearly proscribed sin. The General Medical Council (GMC) 'good practice' series insists we are responsible for the continuous monitoring of our own performance and especially to know our limitations. This has to be progress. The days of have-a-go doctors, including not just surgeons out of their depth but GPs doing procedures, physicians pronouncing judgements and psychiatrists doing strange things they had no authority to do, seem largely to have gone. Now to our peril we veer towards not doing anything without a lawyer's permission, as has been extensively discussed in the medical press.

But the profession has a responsibility to all parties involved to limit the consequences of its nervousness. That there is a personal consequence to lacking confidence is hardly news to many GPs. Anxiety can strike doctors just as the general population, with restless nights or illnesses such as irritable bowel syndrome (IBS) that at least have a partially psychosomatic origin.[8] But the danger for their patient is in misjudging who should be taking full control of the patient's health.

It is unwise, clearly, to over-investigate. GPs are rewarded by society to make judgements with the resources available to them, and to avoid squandering them, yet the patient in front of them seems happiest with more tests, or more interest being taken in them. Well, we all want to be nice. So it is less likely to cause night sweats in the GP if the patient's night sweats are investigated thoroughly, with a view to eliminating TB as a first line. There is evidence that a doctor makes the decision to do 'tests' based only partly on their own knowledge base (or belief in it) but in large measure from intrinsic factors of the doctor's personality, and extrinsic events, like recent publicity.[9,10]

The toughest dilemma is created by the patients who, on the one hand, want certainty, a consumerist one-stop solution, and a world in which the illness can be reliably left with the doctor or nurse to be sorted out and picked up after work that evening like so much dry cleaning. This approach allows the patient to get on with the important things in life and pay the clinician to deal with his or her health. Then, on the other hand, there is the more subtle, complex and realistic view of most illness, which is that it is forever owned by the patient. The doctor is a mere adviser, and secondarily a technician. Many patients will express this to be their own view, but their desire, and possibly their body language, says they want a miracle worker please, to sort it, by tonight.

The unconfident GP either panders to the generally unvoiced desire of the patient to have the doctor totally in control and then finds the potato too hot to handle, or is dismissive and in danger of appearing uncaring. GPs' judgement of where their role is and their confidence in what is possible, and what is not, is the problem. The degree of shared decision making that results is becoming measurable.[11]

So we need our doctors to feel just the right level of confidence in their advice and decision making, perhaps solid at the core but prepared to adapt, listen and change at the edges. It is the intention of this book to define and help guide clinicians towards that.

Decision-making theory

There is a whole discipline of research into medical decision making. It is quite hardgoing to read around this topic because of the unfamiliar jargon used by those in the field. This has originated from psychological research and is directed at solving diagnostic problems for the most part. Initially the research was aimed at looking at how experienced doctors went about solving problems, and having analysed that trying to build this skill explicitly into the medical student curriculum.[10] As a result many modern medical courses have a large element of problem-based learning in which the techniques and principles of cracking a problem (such as 'Mrs Smith is 75 and her knee is swollen and painful') are used throughout. The students work as a group on the issue to great depth and learn to share information, gather it together and formulate ideas and test them.

Moving on from pure problem solving the researchers have looked at how doctors manage in the face of incomplete information or uncertainty, and what reasoning pathways they use. The basic hypothetico-deductive model is the traditionally taught mechanism for medical students in which they have a case with a stack of information and they form hypotheses. A hypothesis will generate predictions and these can be tested so a search for diagnostic, definitive findings is made. A patient presents with a pain in the leg and one suspects (or hypothesises) him or her to have intermittent claudication so therefore he or she should have clinical signs of a poor arterial supply to the foot. A nice warm foot and good pulses make this hypothesis to all intents and purposes invalid but the next hypothesis, perhaps sciatica, can now be tested. Eventually a plan is formed with some degree of confidence and certainty.

But if you look at the experienced doctor, he or she appears to leap to the conclusion by a kind of pattern recognition. It is possible that he or she is just very fast at going through the hypotheses, deductions and tests sequence, which amounts to the same thing, but the strongest theory is that there is a pattern recognition mechanism going on.

The doctor's decision

What is it that runs around a farmyard, is small, brown, feathered, lays eggs and barks?

It's a chicken. You have to ignore the barking.

If you watch a dermatologist at work he or she does the most obvious pattern recognition with the simple visual aid of being able to view the whole problem at once. This looks like a riddle to many students and young doctors: How did they identify this rash so quickly? It is quite demoralising to start learning about skin disease and try to use the hypothetico-deductive method, when in walks the smart dermatologist and gets to the point with a momentary glance.

It seems the skilled diagnostician is adept at spotting the relevant information and assembling it into a pattern to be viewed as a whole. He or she learns to ignore the barking, as it were, whilst not forgetting it entirely in case it becomes necessary, in the light of new evidence in the case, to reconsider. But if the problem is more complex or not amenable to a quick pattern recognition solution then the experienced doctor reverts to the more ponderous student method. It is therefore interesting to speculate on how we develop the pattern recognition ability. Either we learn from previous cases and see similarities or we have a theoretical knowledge, a little nugget of fact that was picked up somewhere and helps us with the pattern.

Using Bayes' theorem,[12] errors creep in with either a failure to form suitable hypotheses in the first place, which is a knowledge issue, or in choosing the 'wrong' information or emphasising the less important details to unbalance the picture. So young doctors will often overestimate the possibility of a rare condition (inappropriate hypothesis), or give undue weight to a slightly odd feature of a case (added information poorly judged), and get to the wrong place. This is explored further in the next chapter.

GPs faced with the volume of cases we see can only cope by pattern-recognising many conditions or situations and not testing the idea too much – but testing it a little. Of course we all make mistakes and commonly this will be from assumptions we make when we think we have seen a familiar pattern. It dawns on us later during the consultation that what we were assuming to be another case of acute bronchitis is actually more like asthma, or the dyspeptic patient actually has something more like IBS. We think to ourselves that it was fortunate that we thought about it again, though actually it is part of our quite rigorous intellectual training to do so. After all, part of the excitement of the job is that we see so many cases that are different patterns of the same thing, or new problems and patterns altogether that require us time and again to go back to first principles of diagnostic thinking and start again.

13

Decision-making aids

What about computer programs that guide the doctor or the patient towards the solution? With the advent of computerisation this was seen as the way general practice might go, with software which ensures that the diagnosis is reached safely and accurately with the careful use of good questions. This has not happened in everyday life partly because of the man who eats newspapers, but also because of a structural reason with the software.

NHS Direct does use decision-support software, and to be fair this is improving all the time. But it is interesting to note that in over two decades of development of this idea there is still no quick computer program to help us. This is because computers essentially use the hypothetico-deductive model (laboriously testing patients with chest pain for anything that might be construed as angina is important to it, whereas the doctor talking on the phone to the anxious-sounding young woman with muscular pain is unlikely to take long to put angina at the bottom of his or her list of possible patterns). They also lack judgement of the overall situation and have a very unsophisticated view of the psycho-social side of illness. The computers play safe in other words, and trudge up to their conclusion wearily if ultimately with some accuracy.

Primary care doctors appear to get there by a different route (though perhaps with equal weariness). This is what we do.

Conclusion

Our judgements and decisions are complex, and the way they are reached is unique to every situation. The public wants us to be certain and confident yet we know this to be inappropriate, and we have to explain that. There is a tendency to nervousness and anxiety in primary care that is worth understanding and analysing. Of course we want to feel good and confident too, and we can improve our confidence as doctors with good communication skills and a strong use of science, yet with some scepticism of the value of evidence-based medicine (EBM) when applied to the patient in front of us.

References

1. Wolfe T. *The Bonfire of the Vanities* London: Picador, 1990.

2. Smith C, Allen J. *Violent Crime in England and Wales 2004* London: Home Office Research, Development and Statistics Directorate, 2005.

3. Leese B, Young R. *Disappearing GPs – is there a recruitment crisis?* Manchester: National Primary Care Research and Development Centre, 1999.

4. Appleton K, House A, Dowell A. A survey of job satisfaction, sources of stress and psychological symptoms amongst GPs in Leeds *British Journal of General Practice* 1998; **48**: 1059–63.

5. Thompson WT, Cupples ME, Sibbert CH, *et al*. The challenge of culture conscience and contract, and GPs' care of their own health *British Medical Journal* 2001; **323**: 728.

6. Grieve S. Measuring morale – does practice area deprivation affect doctors' wellbeing *British Journal of General Practice* 1997; **47**: 547–52.

7. Handysides S. Morale in general practice: is change the problem or the solution? *British Medical Journal* 1994; **308**: 32–4.

8. Winefield H, Murrell T, Clifford J. Sources of occupational stress for Australian GPs and their implications for GP training *Family Practice* 1994; **11**: 413–16.

9. Gruppen L, Wolf FM, Stross JK. Physician practice characteristics and a context for primary care decision making *Academic Medicine* 1990; **65(suppl. 9)**: S9–10.

10. Elstein AS, Schwartz A. Clinical problem solving and diagnostic decision making: selective review of the cognitive literature *British Medical Journal* 2002; **324**: 729–32 [part of a series of five articles].

11. Elwyn G, Edwards A, Wensing M, *et al*. Shared decision making: developing the OPTION scale for measuring patient involvement *Quality and Safety in Health Care* 2003; **12**: 93–9.

12. Gill CJ, Sabin L, Schmid CH. Why clinicians are natural Bayesians *British Medical Journal* 2005; **330**: 1080–3.

CHAPTER 2

A few words about numbers

This section is a brief discussion of the commoner statistical terms and more especially their limitations. A start is made on the issues of communicating risks and assessing the value of numerical data in day-to-day primary care decision making.

That the GP needs to have a good grasp of the statistics of his or her profession to be a confident decision maker is clear. Fighting one's way through the MRCGP and other examinations makes one a transient expert in the field of statistical jargon but somehow, in everyday use, we can lose track of the point of understanding numbers.

Numbers are only occasionally directly available to help with a decision concerning the patient in front of us. We might be able to give statistics on the risks to a woman of using HRT, by using oft-quoted values for the increased incidence of breast cancer after so many years of hormone supplements. But the patient in front of us might have a particular family history, have not breast-fed, be slightly outside the age range in the studies, have had an excess of chest X-rays or whatever, all contributing to alter the risk numbers in her case one way or another. Then she might have a sister who had benign breast cysts, a neighbour who found HRT brilliant, a sexless marriage breaking up, or an embarrassing difficulty swallowing tablets – all of which might influence her perception of the risk, value and practicality of taking the medicine. Our job as advisers to patients cannot be purely evidence based, even where there is apparent evidence to use.[1]

The additional issues of the bias GPs put into their advice, as a result of their previous clinical experience, is discussed in Chapter 6.

In contrast to concordance issues with treatments, some patients seem to accept with notable enthusiasm any suggestion from the GP that the problem might be clarified by means of blood and other tests. A test that to them is likely to give a yes/no answer is perceived as the best way forward, a step away from uncertainty.

The rate of increase of use of investigations by doctors was around 7 per cent per year in the Netherlands in the first years of this century.[2] It is likely to be similar here. This was not matched by a similar improvement in the health of the population, so we can cautiously deduce that quite a lot of tests achieve nothing very much. So why are we doing them? There are of course a number of obvious reasons for this:

- the patient demands it. There is a category of patient who does indeed like the reassurance of the laboratory test, above and beyond the skills of the clinician. The UK GP might be more protected from this tendency than primary care physicians working in even more consumerist societies. But still this does not absolve us all from informing the patients of the value or otherwise of the test and there is evidence that the pressure from patients is more perceived than real[3]

- the practice of defensive medicine, a pure doctor need. Other unspoken doctor needs might include hopeful prevarication (spend time on a test whilst the patient mysteriously gets better) and sheer medical anxiety

- the test is very easy to do. It has been well-shown that if you provide easy access for a new test that hitherto was more awkward to arrange then there is an increased demand for it. This is particularly clear with ultrasound examinations of the abdomen. Nevertheless this does not make these tests invalid and, given that they have little morbidity attached and reasonable sensitivity for conditions we wish to rule out like gallstones, then we should not feel bad about this. CT scans of the head are another example where primary care doctors have been shown to have reasonable skills in picking who should have them, when compared with consultants, even though we have different populations[4]

- the test is arranged to check on a previously unexpected abnormality in another test.

The problem for many doctors is this last category. A biochemical or haematological parameter reference range only means of course that 95 per cent of patients fall within that range. Five per cent of patients will be outside of it, many of whom have no disease and are normal. If a GP bundles off a set of 'routine' bloods on a patient who is, say, 'tired' then there might be approaching 20 values or numbers that return to him or her, of which one at least might be outside the reference range by chance, and without significance. So we all confuse our staff by marking 'normal' or 'no action required' against some results that the computer has highlighted as being 'abnormal'. GPs seem to understand this well and identify the truly abnormal abnormal and act on it. The issue is that in order to identify those significant ones some of the 'erroneously abnormal' ones will be picked up too and so a spiral of more tests begins.

The value of the test

Please try to read this section in one go. The values quoted are for illustration and might not be current. I am certain that this is not new information to you and that you have read it in other forms elsewhere.

It is hard to get the brain into action over the use of statistics for diagnostic tests. We are not an impressively numerate profession. So, to revise: basic diagnostic test performance can be looked at by analysing 'sensitivity' and 'specificity', and, if one has an idea of prevalence, we can measure the 'positive predictive value'.

Sensitivity is the chance of a test being positive when the patient has a disease. So a test with 99 per cent sensitivity means 99 out of 100 people who have the disease will be positive for the test too. If nearly everyone who has the disease has a positive test it means a negative test result is pretty trustworthy, i.e. patients with a negative result are unlikely to have the disease because nearly all diseased patients are positive. Therefore it is useful to have a sensitive test to rule patients OUT (Professor Sacks, evidence-based medicine guru at Oxford, simplifies this to high SeNsitivity rules patients OUT = SNOUT).

It does not tell us whether some other people who do not have the disease are positive for the test too. You can have a very sensitive test that gives lots of false positives amongst all the true positives.

Specificity is the power of the test to be negative if the patient does not have the problem. A 99 per cent-specific test will mean 99 per cent of positives will have the disease – there are few false positives. If nearly all the positives have the disease, then the test is very specific: this is where SPecificity rules patients IN = SPIN. The specificity of a test does not tell us if we can trust a negative result (you need the sensitivity for that). So unless the test is also highly sensitive some patients with negative results might be falsely negative, having the condition despite the negative result. A very specific test ruling patients in is reliable for individual patients with a positive result (they will have the disease), but it doesn't catch everyone with the disease.

No test is 100 per cent sensitive and specific, though some get close. Anyway, as a practical doctor you want to know what importance to place on a positive result – does it mean anything? This is not the only thing you might wish to know but it is important. This is the *positive predictive value*, the proportion of people with a positive test who actually have the disease, and to work this out you need to know the pre-test likelihood of the patient having the disease – the prevalence. This is not the local population's prevalence of the disease, but the prevalence in patients like the one whom you are testing (i.e. similar age, background, hair colour or whatever).

HIV testing is done by double testing – if a sample is screened positive it is not confirmed as positive until tested by another test method as well. The sensitivity of just the first part of the double test is reportedly 100 per cent, so we know that if you have a negative result you do not have HIV even at that stage. The problem comes with a positive result because the specificity of the screening test is 99.8 per cent, which means 0.2 per cent of the population who do not have the disease will nevertheless have shown a positive result. The addition of the second test reduces this to around 0.01 per cent of the population. Using these figures when applied to a population of low-risk patients – the worried well – might initially look reliable. But Gigerenzer, a German statistician and professor of psychology, points out that this is not the case.[5] If the prevalence of HIV in the low-risk population is around 0.01 per cent (true for Germany in the 1990s) then the positive predictive value of an HIV test in this group is only 50 per cent – this is the chance that someone from this group with a positive result actually has the disease.

This is correct. From this data only half the positive results are accurate. Despite a test being 100 per cent sensitive and 99.99 per cent specific, which would look clear cut to most people, 0.01 per cent false positives is the same rate as the prevalence or true positives.

The point of this exercise is to illustrate that looking at these figures is rather mind blowing and just when you thought you had grasped it you get a dizzy turn.

Another simpler way of understanding these numbers is to abandon probabilities and percentages, and talk in terms of absolute numbers and frequencies.

Imagine 10,000 low-risk people all having an HIV test. We know that 1 of the 10,000 is likely to have the disease because the prevalence of it is 0.01 per cent or 1 in 10,000. The test is 100 per cent sensitive so everyone who has the disease has a positive test, and thus this one person will have a positive test. Unfortunately the test is only 99.99 per cent specific so one poor person in 10,000 has a positive test too, despite not having the disease. There are therefore two people with positive tests but only one of them has the disease. The positive predictive value is therefore only 1 in 2.

If you do this for a population at significant risk then the results are less scary. If the prevalence is 1 per cent then, of our 10,000 patients, 100 will have the disease and they are all going to have a positive test. One other will have a falsely positive test, and so 100/101 is the new positive predictive value.

How can a test be positive despite being double-checked and looked at by two methods? This rare event is more often due to data errors, e.g. wrong labelling of the sample, mixing of the results on a computer database or transcription errors, than to an assay problem. So the answer for our low-risk patient who has a positive result is to have a new sample tested, ideally by a different lab and method, before coming to any conclusions about his or her future.

For a GP the difficulty is that the decision to do a test is not usually made in the knowledge of recent specificity, sensitivity and prevalence data, and even if it is then the data might not apply to the population he or she is testing, i.e. the test performance changes with the population and we simply cannot factor in all the parameters.

So what to do? The prudent GP will be aware to an extent of the value of many tests. For instance the emergency electrocardiogram (ECG) beloved of ambulance crews does not have an acceptable sensitivity for ruling out a myocardial infarction (MI) in patients with chest pain; it is only around 90 per cent sensitive. It might be reasonably specific, also at around 90 per cent – those with abnormal ECGs are highly likely to have disease, but too many patients having an MI have a normal ECG.

The D-dimer test is sensitive enough to help eliminate patients with a possible deep-vein thrombosis (DVT) in that if there is a DVT the result is nearly always raised, but as there are many other causes of a raised D-dimer a positive result is unhelpful in making the diagnosis.

From time to time other tests are devised and investigated. There is a great need for a clear, simple test for heart failure, for instance. For a while a test called BNP (beta-type natriuretic peptide) was touted as a diagnostic test since it showed reasonable results in that the patients with heart failure in the initial studies were positive and the ones with normal hearts were negative. The sensitivity figures looked reasonable. But when the test was used on primary care patients, not those with known heart failure (as judged by echocardiography) but those with *suspected* disease from the clinical picture, it turned out that the test was far less discriminatory. The sensitivity of the test dropped in part because the population from primary care included so many others without heart failure (although they had problems that justified looking for it) rather than those with known disease versus those known to be completely free of it. The original investigators also placed their 'cut-off' point for the test being abnormal in an ideal position on the scale to maximise the apparent performance of the test. When used independently in other studies this cut-off gave much worse reliability.

Poorly sensitive and specific tests

We therefore understand that tests are inadequate in that they do not, for the patient in front of you, tell you, necessarily, what is happening. But clinical decision making is based on numerous bits of unreliable data, from the history and examination, as well as through to our beloved tests. If the information is taken as a whole, yet in sequence, then the final conclusion can be more certain.

Bayes, an eighteenth-century mathematician-vicar (remembered more for his statistics than his theology), said that the pre-test odds of a hypothesis being true could be multiplied by a formula, the 'likelihood ratio', to give post-test odds.[6] This 'likelihood ratio' is a function of the sensitivity and specificity of a given test. The post-test odds become the pre-test odds when the next test is brought in, and so on. It all works, apparently, so long as the tests are unrelated. Some of the tests we apply to our patient are bits of history (does it hurt when the patient coughs?) or examination (is the patient's throat red?) that can be considered part of this process, as well as a formal 'test'.

In clinical terms at some point we think of all the information we get about a patient and form not only a hypothesis but also an idea of the likelihood of it being true. So, does this young man with chest pain have ischaemic heart disease? How can we test this and how far can we go before we consider it proven or disproven? It has been said that, as diagnosticians, we are mostly Bayesian thinkers. The process is instinctive to doctors, but it is reassuring that the mathematicians can put numbers and formulae to it.

The numerate GP and the puzzled patient

The decisive doctor has to base his or her confidence on something, and there are some certainties we can identify, like the safety of childhood vaccines and the need for aspirin in ischaemic heart disease (yet even these have little exclusions). Given that this level of confidence is only available for the minority of decisions we have to make, we rely on the numbers to inform rather than to decide, and this is why we need to understand the level of trustworthiness of the proposed action, whether to test or give a treatment. We then have to impart this to the patient who, confusingly, has a different angle on this from us.[7]

Explaining numbers is difficult but one has no hope unless one understands them oneself. This is why I have tediously gone on about evaluating the performance of tests. There is a whole literature on explaining risks and how doctors should try to change their language to get a better understanding across to the patient. Remember we are trying to achieve more confident decision making by getting patients to take more responsibility for the outcome of the consultation, and they need to understand the figures to do that.

As a gross generalisation, patients do not understand

1. percentages (e.g. there is a 5 per cent rate of wound infection) especially if comparing them

2. vague verbal cues like 'high risk', 'common' and 'likely'

3. probabilities (e.g. you have a 1 in 250 chance of dying from the operation).

Experts in communicating risk, like John Paling, find that patients understand numbers expressed as frequencies instead. So – instead of saying the odds of getting breast cancer rise from 1 in 67 to 1 in 53 in a five-year period if a woman takes HRT – it is easier to say

> Out of 1000 women aged 50–69 over five years, 15 will get breast cancer. If they all took HRT then 19 will develop the disease.

The patient can then immediately understand the scale of the risk.

The verbal odds

Several authorities have suggested that if we want to avoid frequencies or don't know the exact number, but also want to avoid odds to describe risk, we should at least be consistent with our words. One suggestion (from Paling) is as follows:

Doctor term	Equates to
Very High Risk	1 in 1 to 1 in 10
High Risk	1 in 10 to 1 in 100
Moderate	1 in 100 to 1 in 1000
Low	1 in 1000 to 1 in 10,000
Very Low	1 in 10,000 to 1 in 100,000
Minimal	1 in 100,000 to 1 in 1,000,000
Effectively Zero	1 in 1,000,000 or less

I think for UK GPs this works except that for 'effectively zero' say 'zero'.

The worst confusion arises from a discussion using relative risks. This drug company marketing ploy should never be used for discussion with patients. For example, the Roche drug Herceptin was said by the BBC and others to 'halve the chances of the disease recurring in early-stage breast cancer'. This figure was based on a drug company study of 1694 carefully selected women.[8] Results indicated a 17.2 per cent chance of recurrence at a year in the untreated group compared with a 9.4 per cent chance in the treated group. About 8.5 per cent stopped the drug because of problems (and in another US trial some 18.5 per cent stopped the drug). Some had significant cardiac problems that seemed related to the treatment. Publicity suggested this drug was wonderful, but the study results suggested that only 7.8 per cent (or 1 in 13) benefited from the treatment, and a similar number suffered significant adverse reactions, even in a very carefully selected group. If patient survival is prolonged – and it is not possible to equate one-year recurrence figures with longer-term survival – then the cost per life saved (by the drug company's own figures) was around half a million pounds and actual experience is likely to be worse than that. It is now licensed for this group of patients. But I suppose that the BBC version was true, just seriously short of the whole truth.

The other advice for doctors explaining risks and chances is to use visual aids. If you take a piece of paper with 1000 icons representing people and mark the ones at risk of whatever – say the 15 out of a 1000 who will get breast cancer – then the additional ones who get it on HRT are easily visualised. This is in Paling's book along with other visual aids (see Figures 2.1 and 2.2 overleaf).[7]

Conclusion

GPs need to aspire to occasional numeracy and apply it where they can. If well informed, this might discourage over-investigation and help in sharing decision making. GPs will not use numbers at every consultation, but, when they do, they must explain them clearly through the techniques of using frequencies and the pictorial representations alluded to.

References

1. Slowther A. The ethics of evidence based medicine in a primary care setting *Journal of Medical Ethics* 2004; **30**: 151–5.

2. Winkens R, Dinant G. Rational, cost effective use of investigations in clinical practice *British Medical Journal* 2002; **324**: 783–5.

3. Little P, Dorward M, Warner G, *et al*. Importance of patient pressure and perceived pressure and perceived medical need for investigations referral and prescribing in primary care: nested observational study *British Medical Journal* 2004; **328**: 444–6 plus comment p. 416.

4. Goadsby PJ. To scan or not to scan in headache *British Medical Journal* 2004; **324**: 469–70.

5. Gigerenzer G. *Reckoning with Risk* London: Penguin, 2002.

6. Gill CJ, Sabin L, Schmid CH. Why clinicians are natural Bayesians *British Medical Journal* 2005; **330**: 1080–3.

7. Paling J. *Helping Patients Understand Risk* Gainesville, FL: The Risk Communication Institute, 2006, www.riskcomm.com [accessed July 2008].

8. Figures as issued on press release, June 2006. Some detailed data published in Gonzalez-Angulo AF, Hortobagyi AM, Esteva GN, *et al*. Adjuvant therapy with trastuzumab for HER-2/neu-positive breast cancer *Oncologist* 2006; **11**: 857–67.

Figure 2.1: The Paling palette

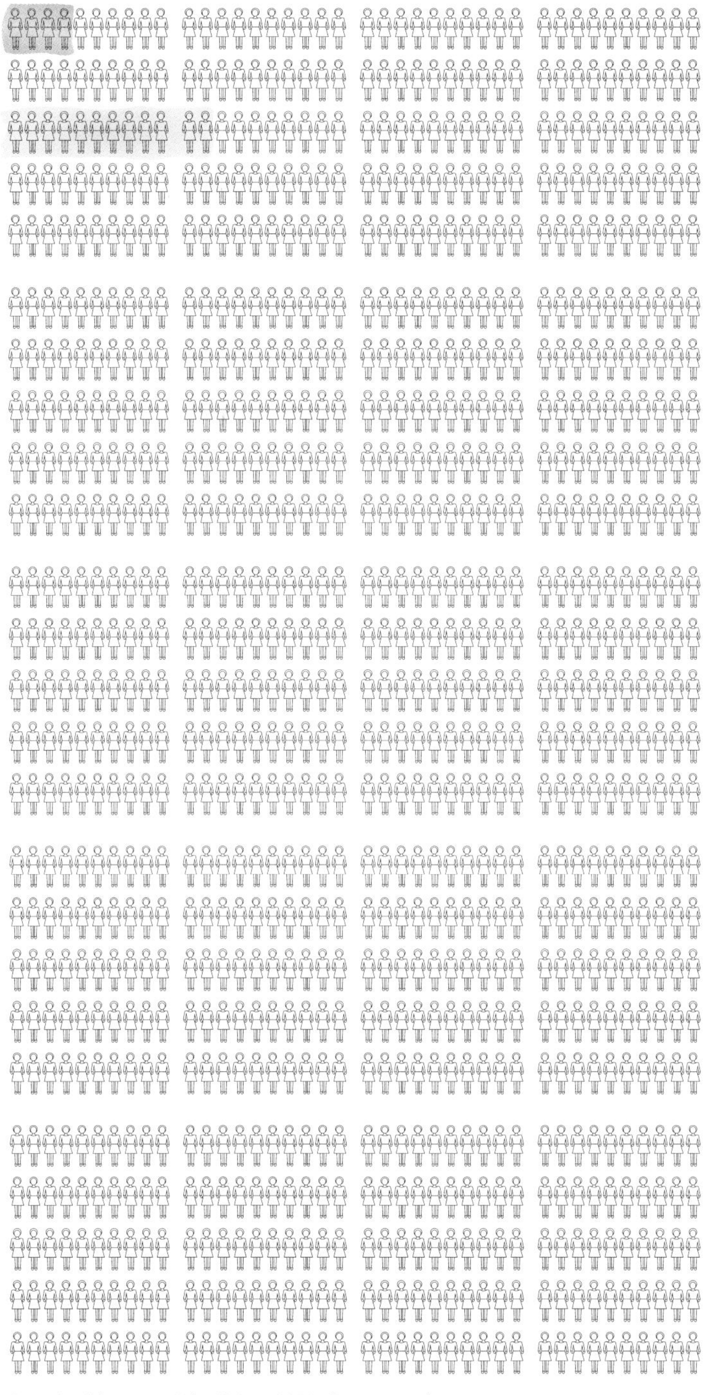

Visual aid format © John Paling 2000. See www.riskcomm.com.

Figure 2.2: The Paling perspective scale

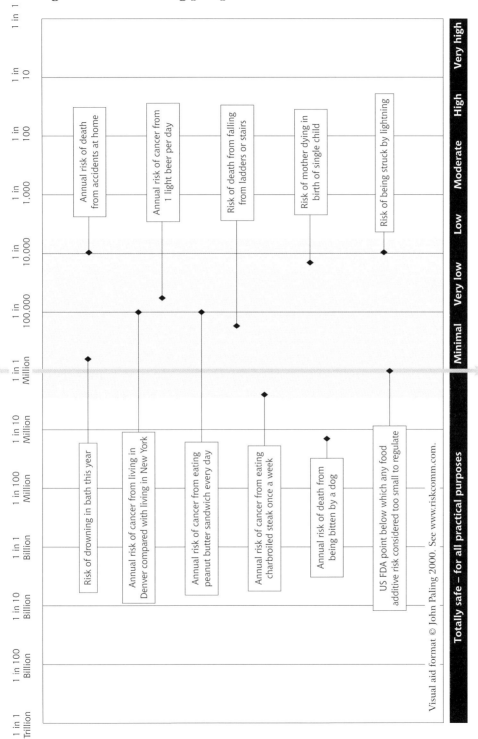

Visual aid format © John Paling 2000. See www.riskcomm.com.

CHAPTER 3

What am I here for?

This chapter is a discussion of the modern GP's role, deconstructing it into a set of challenges and goals in the consultation. The emphasis is to help the doctor be realistic yet valued, not least by him or herself. Using numerous clinical examples the intention is to help doctors who are frustrated by their uncertainty and perceived ineffectiveness to re-evaluate their importance to the patient.

A politician's career can succeed or fail on the publication from time to time of the number of clinicians employed within the NHS. Naturally, various statistical devices are used to put the best looking numbers on the front of the press release – counting heads rather than whole time equivalents, counting outputs from training rather than actual real live working doctors and nurses, and so on. This is to be expected and is not unreasonable in a democracy, I may add, so long as the true detail is also available. But the underlying assumption that the very existence of extra clinicians is a Good Thing is politically sacrosanct. There might be a debate at a political level around shifting work from one group to another – typically from junior doctors to senior nurses, or from secondary to primary care doctors – but the received wisdom is nevertheless that we clinicians are here as a necessary force for good in society. To question whether doctors and nurses are helpful is like asking if food is an important commodity. It is a stupid question and requires a truly rebellious social and medical commentator such as Illich to stir us into thinking about it.[1]

Yet any half-educated doctor knows that most substantive health gains are the result of greater wealth and its distribution rather than the activities of the healthcare industry. There is little or no correlation between healthcare spending in the Western world and population health. But some correlation is found between the markers of health, like perinatal mortality and the level of inequality within a society. Logically our politician, who stands or falls on the count of doctors and nurses, should be accountable differently. Health can be measured in various proxy ways, and since it parallels socio-economic conditions the voters ought, in a reasonable debate, to be shown that link. Vote for me and you are less likely to have a heart attack! All rather unlikely, and the simplistic solution of employing and counting lots of clever health experts like us is the preferred if disingenuous measure of health. It might be, of course, that there are benefits to the GPs, consultants and other clinical staff in colluding with this false impression, but as I am determined not to be cynical this line of argument will, for the moment at least, stop here.

Although a patient might be hopelessly grateful for being cured of his or her ills, in private doctors know that nature (whatever that is) should be awarded most of the credit. Much of the time we doctors, especially in primary care, are merely well-informed bystanders. Exceptions to this rule abound, of course. Patients who have had a technical procedure like a minor operation might well have cause to thank the technical team, starting with the diagnosing GP. However, at a deeper level their susceptibility to illness in the first place is related to their socio-economic position, genetics, lifestyle and environment. The healing process after a procedure is 'nature', and one of the largest factors influencing the course of the patient's recovery is his or her 'constitution'. We know patients with pneumonia are statistically more likely to have a good outcome if they are given antibiotics, but a number will succumb despite them, while others will recover untreated (though patients are unlikely to believe this). The differences between those who do well and those who don't is therefore much more than whether they have had the drug, but these differences are intrinsic. We do not necessarily understand them, let alone influence them, and yet we take the credit for a good result.

And in some cases whether they really needed the treatment or whether the procedure was truly to benefit them, or they were merely sold it, is certainly an issue for legitimate debate, albeit less so in a socialised medical system like the NHS. The debate about when tests and procedures are useful is complicated and emotive. Many GPs would argue that we do too much and cite the various unwelcome pressures on us. Sometimes we too persuade patients in good faith to have an intervention because of our latest enthusiasms, only to find later on evidence that the patient's outcome was unaffected, and we might even feel guilty. In private medical systems patients are often encouraged to have interventions of uncertain value (like an 'annual physical') and we might or might not feel guilty there too: there is clear evidence that the volume of surgery seemingly indicated in an area is more closely linked to the number of surgeons available than the health of the population they serve. But then perhaps subjective measures like the patient feeling better for seeing a particular doctor ought to be enough to warrant the work.

Nevertheless the argument is not that the doctor is invariably useless in affecting outcomes, merely that the clinician in charge might not actually be in a position to do a lot – and yet is credited with such power. And, being human, rather enjoys the credit.

This is not yet doing a lot for clinical self-confidence.

To even ask the question 'What am I here for?' betrays an uncertainty that might seem unhelpful. It sounds like a question a management consultant (picture him – young, male, conservative dresser but with red socks) might ask on a team away-day as an 'original' challenge to think through the purpose and function of some individual's role. But, indeed, it is important because if the question seems silly then perhaps that means it is tough. If it is difficult then perhaps we don't want to face the answer. Especially if the gut instinct, as above, is to joke self-effacingly 'not a lot'.

There is a dichotomy between this politician-fed public faith and trust in us as crucial members of society and our own confidence in what we can actually do. The status we are given might feel unearned at times, especially as at other times GPs seem to be viewed as simplistic referral agencies happy just to 'Choose and Book' our cases.

In considering what we are here for, there seems a case for first asking what we want. Not just what the patient wants. Studies of many GP consultations assume, for instance, that the doctor is acting altruistically on the patient's behalf and that a good outcome for the patient is a good outcome for the doctor too.

Perhaps this is naïve.

The truth is that our actions are a compromise between our personal needs, the patient's expressed wants and his or her objective needs – if these can be identified. A useful discussion of this by Gothill, a London academic GP, developed the idea of the doctor's internal audience that he or she is trying to please.[2] Not the doctor's material comfort, especially, but his or her inner satisfaction – and (for the moment) never mind the patient. This internal audience might be pleased easily, perhaps content simply to trundle along, avoiding complaints and criticisms. On the other hand the internal audience might be a real 'mother-in-law type' of critic who has to be fed steadily with reassurances and pleasantries, and yet does little to acknowledge positive work. (This concept of an internal nagging machine is alarming but we do hope to switch it off!) So taking the logic of this further Gothill concludes that being patient centred is where the internal audience is more like a patient, and being clinician centred is more like having an internal colleague.

Now we know that to be patient centred is close to being saintly and a goal towards which we must all strive. Sometimes it seems only those born with some mysterious and divinely inspired genetic ability can really be truly patient centred all the time. But we can also look at it simply as a counterweight to our usual and protective tendency to be clinician centred, which we can and must learn to switch on when appropriate.[3] For we do not always have to look at altruism as a good thing in itself, because it might only be good for one of the parties involved. The sum total of human happiness might have gone up, at considerable cost to the clinician, but there might be another way that is cheaper. First the GP has to be comfortable with what he or she is there for.

Gift horses and the role into which we are driven

It feels mean to question gifts and hint that they are not as freely given as one might like to think. Nevertheless it is fun to consider the matter and speculate on the patients' motives.

As a medical student, I realised the power game involved when a child psychiatrist from whose firm I was learning about mental health received a well-wrapped Christmas gift of a large cigar from an encopretic child. This was of course only just short of actually sending a stool through the post and the child had not only expressed defiance to him – 'I can place my stool anywhere I wish' – but also must have got the parent to collude by purchasing and posting it. This sad present presumably heralded a poor prognosis.

On a more mundane level patients who have a long-term relationship with their GP will often try to move from being a patient to being a friend. This might involve a direct gift (triggering a rush of patronising jollity in the Christmas medical journals). Or more insidiously, perhaps, by finding out the ages and names of one's children and sending the over-privileged darlings a token present, or occasionally more. Most GPs and doctors who have a long-term relationship with patients have experienced this. This change is not comfortable. We like to set the boundaries and not have them moved, for when they are we feel rather lost. What are we supposed to do when the gift giver seems to hint for a little extra service, like being seen outside normal appointment times, or preferential treatment of some kind? Many patients would like this, and indeed ask for better service, but for reasons of practicality we have to restrict how flexible we can be. Giving a gift seems to increase the guilt felt by the GP as they decline to treat the patient differently from others – sometimes there is a feeling one should allow some sort of tit for tat (the tat, generally, coming from the patient).

Slightly more subtly, patients are also aware that it is in their interests that we like them, so that we listen better, giving thought and an earlier follow-up to their case without a specific request.

One old lady who had considerable medical problems but was, to use a politically incorrect phrase, demanding, would nevertheless always send the visiting doctor or nurse away with a foil-wrapped sponge cake. In the early years these were quite tasty but as time went on and her health declined, so did the quality of her cakes until they were generally quite inedible. Sometimes they were merely stale, while at other times they showed more signs of life than she did. Be reassured that, professional to the end, we maintained her care until she entered a distant nursing home.

It really is time to redress the balance from the negativity, gloom and hopeless-ness presented so far.

May I present a crude list of what use front-line doctors really are to the rest of the world? This might at first seem like a startling glimpse of the obvious, but in a chapter about what one is here for it is essential. Rather than the generalisation that our duty is the relief of suffering – which in its broadest sense is what most work is about – we can try to break it down:

- curing people (just occasionally)
- being a listener
- ensuring accuracy of understanding about the past
- giving information about the present
- giving information about the future
- advising on risky behaviours
- advising on options available, including risk assessments
- advising on pain and relief of other symptoms
- acting as health police and advising authorities
- co-ordinating care
- being a comforter
- comforting the relatives.

All of which makes us pretty important.

Curing people

Sadly, the true cure is a rare pleasure for most of us. I can rid someone of their ear wax, or with drugs lift their depression, but both have a habit of returning. The mum who explains to the child that the 'doctor is going to make you better' is usually misinformed, although obviously we will do our best. It's actually quite hard to think of cures we give that don't involve the use of anti-infective treat-ments. We might have a principle hand in sorting out the odd case of headache, bereavement reaction, incontinence or minor injury.

If we set a purist standard of cure as the return of the patient to their pre-disease state, then even sending patients for 'curative' operations like, say, a hysterec-tomy for early endometrial carcinoma, or a new hip, leaves scars both physical and mental. Patients are changed by the experience of disease from then on, so a full return as if nothing had happened is only likely for minor conditions and those, for the most part, are self-limiting rather than are cured by us.

We should soften the definition of cure to where a patient has a significant ill-ness, the course of which is stopped or dramatically slowed by our actions – so the patient lives a lot longer or in greater comfort than would otherwise have

29

happened. Many chronic diseases well-suited to primary care long-term management like diabetes, osteoarthritis, ischaemic heart disease and long-term mental illness are in this group. Examples of success here, however, will have involved teams of people and it is therefore wrong for the GP to take sole credit for this 'cure', though they will have had a central, leadership role.

There are exceptions to this and with an effort I can drag up some examples but I contend that most GPs spend only a minority of their time on actually curing people. *What many of us have had the happy experience of doing is being the one who set the ball rolling, who sent the patient to the team who intervened. Or even heading the team who did the intervention, dramatically averting catastrophe. This is one of the core satisfactions of the job, but it is not curing.*

Being a listener

The value of listening to the patient properly cannot of course be underestimated no matter what one's field of medicine is.[*] Much of the communication skills literature is devoted to training us as listeners. But it is vital that all GPs, especially indecisive ones, understand how they are valued by patients as intelligent, important people prepared to give time to listening. The patient might well not understand, let alone articulate, that being listened to is what they need and are getting, but they do appreciate that they feel better for the process.

There seems an issue of maturity here. The registrar or newly qualified GP might well have a sound theoretical belief in the value of listening but he or she still yearns to be getting on with the doing, the relieving, sometimes the curing. *It takes experience to discover that for many patients there is no better 'doing', relieving and even sometimes curing than controlled listening. That listening, far from being what you do when you can't do anything else, is a first-line prime intervention.* An issue of culture complicates this. In many parts of the world, including South Asia, the doctor's role is more respected if he or she sticks to therapeutics, interventions and procedures. The patient who wants a sympathetic listener goes elsewhere. The doctor in Bangladesh, say, deeply sympathetic to the patient's plight, might choose not to show it for fear of losing the confidence of the patient. Herein lies many a confused consultation and so it is important for GPs to understand the culture within which they work, and to pitch their approach correctly.

Ensuring accuracy of understanding about the past

This role might be split into ensuring that patients understand the origin of their current problem and checking they know what their entire list of previous medical encounters and mishaps actually means.

A fascinating glimpse of how patients think is frequently heard when they start the history from a point in time where they perceive their immediate problems began. 'I fell over in the garden last year and then when my chest hurt last week I thought that was it, making it, you know, hard to breathe, though I knew it wasn't

---

[*] An exception might be pathology.

too bad because I wasn't coughing anything up, well any blood or anything you know....' Juxtaposed events create trains of thought that confuse us all. Naturally it is the doctor's role (usually) to disabuse such theories, though humility demands that the patient is given serious attention. After all, we have all been caught out with unlikely tales that turned out to be true, and, even when the patient's ideas of what happened are implausible, we might not have a better theory. So helping patients to understand the past might challenge their ideas of causation and leave them uncertain, but it is still better than colluding with an error. Usually. The empowerment of the patient, which the modern GP heartily promotes, starts with making sure they have the facts straight.

However, it is beholden on the doctor to try not to ascribe anything they can't explain as 'stress', 'a virus' or 'arthritis' in the absence of any evidence. This can be tricky when the patient insists on an explanation, but the skilled GP should handle it without being disingenuous.

Assuming we possess their medical history, though, it is frequently vital that we ensure patients grasp this too. The 1991 legislation giving access to medical records, and the more recent Data Protection Acts, are little used by patients and seem of more value for lawyers to browse and cackle over. This is a shame, as a better relationship ensues when we encourage patients to understand their medical history. We all want the patient to know exactly what operation he or she had, but how very often do we find patients with surgical scars that they cannot explain, or explain fully. One wonders if too little time was spent at the time by the medical staff, or too little went in because of technical jargon or simply too much information. Whatever the reason where we have concrete information about a patient's medical history he or she is grateful for our role in explaining it. And then he or she is more likely to take control.

Giving information about the present

At last, a role for the GP to use all that long expensive training dishing out a summarised and succinct expert explanation of the situation as he or she sees it. It is often a difficult, challenging part of the doctor's role whether the information given is sad or happy news.

Although, as in all medical fields, there is also the mundane and repetitive case with which we have to deal. The patient feels that he or she is an individual with (insert diagnosis here) but it is only human for the doctor or nurse to slot him or her into membership of a group all of whom have (whatever). We find ourselves with well-tuned homilies on whatever our expertise is – explaining the back pain, the endoscopy, the menopause, the blood test. It feels like a macro-button, which gets pressed and then out comes the whole paragraph, unwrapped from the GP's consciousness, and ready for minor individual adjustments as needed. This might well feel dull, and since it is unexciting to us then it's probably pretty boring to the patient too. Yet to the patient there are few more important moments in life. It is on this that the family will want to quiz him or her when the patient returns home: 'What did he or she say?'

Doctors from time to time remark that a particular patient is a poor historian. This sad phrase contains an irony in that, in the transfer of factual information and feelings from patient to doctor, it is the doctor who is the historian. The patient is the witness. Now it is fair to say some patients are clearer-minded witnesses than others, and that it is much easier to be the historian in some situations than others. What seems less variable is that patients are rarely trained listeners and so able to guide the clinician in giving information back to them. Especially as the feelings part will often dominate the factual section. So there is a wealth of depressing research showing how hard it is successfully to give clear information to a patient in any quantity, at least at one sitting. Surely then, this vital role for GPs is also one of our challenges, to be seen as difficult rather than drab.

Giving information about the future

The society that pays us demands foreknowledge, definite predictions, and is far from reasonable with us about our uncertainties. We know something about statistics and therefore find them even less trustworthy than the patient does, yet they are all we have. As the population gets more sophisticated and as we move into a more evidence-based style of practice we can be more confident in our predictions. One of the important skills the GP has is in knowing where useful evidence is about prognosis as well as management and being able to evaluate it (or, failing that, knowing a man who does). We can allow patients to plan, albeit with all kinds of caveats. Time and again, where patients have been prepared to say what image they had of their health, they have started with an inaccurate and frightening view, worse even than we thought. We might think we have bad news, yet it can make them feel better. A classic example is glandular fever (or infectious mononucleosis), which commonly carries an expectation that it will last a year – but more than 90 per cent of patients recover inside a couple of months. This knowledge alone helps people to recover. Evidence for this particularly comes from studies of chronic fatigue syndrome showing that those who believe they have a bad prognosis duly have their prophecy fulfilled.[4]

So, even if we cannot promise they won't be run over by a bus tomorrow, we have considerable powers of prediction that, carefully used, are greatly valued.

Advising on risky behaviours

That the information on smoking, alcohol, unprotected sex and whatever the current food scare might be is so easily and widely ignored seems to be either proof of our failure, or proof of the indomitable human spirit in the face of risk. Yet, on the other hand, we take pride in trials which show that brief interventions from a GP and possibly other clinicians can trigger 2 per cent of patients into quitting smoking. A more autonomous approach would be to look at how accurately smokers and others estimate the personal risk they choose to take. One might argue that the anxious GP worries about the 98 per cent who ignore his or her sound advice, but the confident one sees his or her role as merely ensuring that as many as possible realise that smoking is not somehow safe in their case. The first adviser is almost hurt by the addict's weak response, as if the consequences were his or her own burden.

Here again it is our role to explain that the risks of smoking are clear and severe, whereas the risk of whatever is presently preoccupying the papers is generally a theory, mere conjecture and mathematically unsound. The old joke about the patient who kept reading that smoking was bad for him and so decided to give up reading is based on truth and we have to challenge the tendency to equate risks and then dismiss the lot.

Advising on options available, including risk assessments

If we accept the premise that in most clinical interactions there is no simple cure, a solitary path from which it would be madness to stray, then there are options. To the front-line doctor some are more attractive than others for reasons of practicality, empathy, or perhaps a recent paper he or she has read. Options tend to come with a recommendation and it might all be very complicated.

A fine example from another field of medicine is the change in tone used by modern orthopaedic surgeons. From 'I have decided to do a hip replacement' – *circa* 1975 – to 'We have discussed benefits and the risks (including sepsis, joint failure, pulmonary embolism and anaesthetic risks) and I would think that a hip replacement would be very helpful. The patient is thinking about it and will let me know.' The surgeon has a good evidence base to make his or her recommendation but wisely ducks the responsibility of the final decision; informed consent is a confidence-building concept. The manner in which the risk of each option is discussed is however open to criticism.

Less clear-cut advice is not going to be so much evidence- as judgement-based. We might advise submitting the old lady with mild weight loss to investigation or we might advise waiting; less seriously we might consider offering steroid tablets for, say, aphthous ulcers, but the thought might cross the GP's mind to keep quiet about it. Here it is harder to explore the risks for an individual case, and we have to do our best in the absence of firm data. Here, above all, the GP has to learn to come clean: withholding possible options merely because the doctor, without more than a gut feeling, does not judge them best is liable to go wrong when the patient checks the internet. The doctor is an adviser, not a parent.

Advising on pain and relief of other symptoms

That this is our prime role, the securing of the best outcome in the circumstances by the use of whatever psychological, chemical and technical wizardry we can, is clear. Good communication between patient and the clinician is obviously a part of this.

In some ways, unfortunately, it is inevitable that the patient will seek other sources of trusted information. So we find the neighbour's aunt's advice, the internet, his or her previous experience and the leaflets in the packets of drugs all given an authority and trust that we don't agree with. But remember the patient's symptoms are going to be eased, or not, by a combination of factors, only one of which is whether the expert advice is actually followed. The decision whether to follow that advice is complex, and part of the game is for the doctor to make it safe for the patient to voice the other influences playing on him or her. This is explored later but it is worth remembering that the patient might have a point.[*]

Acting as health police and advising authorities

There is a dreadful term, 'health fascist', used in media discussions since the late 1990s by otherwise intelligent journalists objecting to the latest medical advice on a healthy lifestyle. That they misrepresented whatever that advice said in the first place was common, and that they placed undue weight on it, invariable. So we had 'scares' about coloured Smarties, alco-pops, Chinese and herbal remedies, coloured toilet paper, etc. Shocking, though, was the gross misuse of this term 'fascism', which is a particularly important evil for all humanity to understand. Used in the context of benign health advice equating doctors (generally) with totalitarian police demonstrates how fearsome such advice must be. Or how badly we handled it.

But the GP's duty is not only to the patient in front of him or her; it also includes the folk in the street, the general public, the taxpayer. The ethics of breaching confidentiality in the case of the epileptic patient who continues to drive illegally are clear. A bit less clear might be the pressure genito-urinary clinics apply on patients to reveal sexual contacts (in Sweden for instance this is considered a police matter). Worries around child abuse are notoriously hard to judge, where a balance of rights and responsibilities is sought. Suspicions about corruption or poor performance by a colleague might present the doctor with a dilemma for which they feel not only untrained but also unsupported, either by colleagues or an ethical framework.

Some US hospitals have tried employing a philosopher to help sort out ethical issues, which often involve a conflict between the role of patient advocate and public protector.

Somebody ultimately at some level has to ration care, especially in an age of newly introduced drugs that give at best modest benefits and often less, yet at astonishing costs (an example being beta interferon). This is fascinating but in practice quite unenviable; the decision on the use of resources ought ideally to be political and managerial rather than that of the healthcare professions. We have elaborate mechanisms for deciding what resource is available, like Primary Care Organisations (PCOs), hospital boards, the National Institute for Health and Clinical Excellence (NICE) and general elections. The jobbing GP has a duty to work within these confines and notify the relevant mechanisms when they are unacceptable, and should feel confident that this is what is expected of him or her. The core of this is the relationship with the management and that in turn works by mutual respect; a concept well worth trying out.

---

[*] However, the patient bearing a wad of internet printouts does start at a social disadvantage and somehow there should be a gentle campaign to teach patients to keep their internet sources to themselves or be more tactful with their advisers.

Returning to the role of pure patient advocate, it is of course a duty of GPs to give information, where properly consented, to third parties like insurance companies. Slightly more difficult is giving information to government agencies like the benefits agency – but here one has to understand the part one plays. To give factual data, as completely as possible, in the patient's interest, is a concept lawyers find easier than doctors. The GP is being asked to support the case for housing or a benefit rather than judge it, so the remit is only to give information to that end. Relief arrives with the knowledge that the agency to which one writes (the council, the Department of Social Security, etc.) usually understands this role. Its decision is based on that perception – it alone is responsible for deciding benefit levels, housing, etc. and not the author of the medical report, whatever the recommendation.

Co-ordinating care

The senior nurse on the ward might seem to epitomise the role of co-ordinator, badgering the various professionals involved, or who should be involved, into committing themselves into the package of care the patient warrants either as inpatient or on discharge. This might well become a very wide team depending on the situation. But in the increasingly complex care of patients in the community this forever-on-the-phone role has become entrenched in the GP's job description as well.

The leadership of the team actually delivering care at any one point in the patient's pathway might move, although it is too often the case that the most senior doctor assumes the role, whether appropriate or not. That the team exists at all, rather than a command and control structure, might be news to some within it. It seems clinicians (whatever their backgrounds) are best at doing the co-ordinating and liaising rather than only the caring; it is not something easily delegated to non-clinical managers. This is not because they are good at paperwork but because they are sound at communicating and experienced at assessing and even negotiating. Therefore the role of the GP is often to set up the framework for the patient's care by using administrative staff (secretarial, not managers) to sort the details out afterwards since, almost certainly, the secretary is paid less than the GP.

Being a comforter

That it is inevitable that we spend much of our time dealing with situations that are impossible, deteriorating and hopeless, where all that is on offer is a feeble sympathy, might seem to be a miserable truth; it need not be.[5]

It is the phrase 'dealing with situations' that needs a deeper understanding. A doctor's duty is to take responsibility for his or her advice, and for his or her actions. GPs are responsible for limiting their involvement to those areas where they possess expertise and competence, unless in the role of a supervised learner. They also have to be responsible for assessing the patients' expectations and keeping them appropriate (or at least explaining the professional view of what might be feasible). GPs might be tempted to consider that they have to 'deal' somehow with whatever is presented to them, lest they appear inadequate. But although GPs strive to maximise the boundaries of their expertise, they need to be comfortable staying within them. And how do we define 'situation' when the word conjures up not so much a medical model of a purely health crisis but a complete psycho-social and physical mess: depressingly short of simple curative interventions. A palliative case is not the only such 'situation'.

So here we have a category of clinician–patient interactions that might be beyond giving advice, for little will help, and possibly beyond structured, professional listening. The GP might find him or herself in the manner of a neighbour, a friend whose actions are of little use but whose presence is valued nevertheless. It is a messy relationship, full of baggage and sometimes not quite honest, because to extinguish hope is of course unwise. To cope with this an experienced doctor tries not to be defensive; and finds it is not at all easy.

And the wise one knows that he or she too needs support, if not now then in due course.

Comforting the relatives

This duty is so easily avoided and occasionally this is the best option. Often, though, the conflicts between the patient's and the family's expectations are fascinating and revealing. If the patient is to be treated holistically then the oily dynamics of the family are involved somewhere. The 'family' of a patient might well mean informal carers, like neighbours, pastoral or church workers, or even work colleagues, sometimes more important to our patient than his or her immediate blood relations (and therein lies a story we feel).

A GP is comfortable with the rules of confidentiality even when he or she faces apparently difficult dilemmas and he or she finds that by far the majority of patients understand them too. Involving the relatives is then another patient choice and its pros and cons, probably unrevealed to the doctor, weighed up internally and a verdict given.

This plan works fine when the patient is alive and competent. When the patient is not competent and the doctor is in a parental, controlling role then often the issues are simpler. Following a death, as usual, matters might be more complicated because one does not know what was said or intended to be said, but the relative might well have a need to know, if only for his or her own grieving process. Some stretching of the rules of confidentiality can be best, not least if it relieves further pain.

Conclusion

This chapter tries to break down the job of a primary care clinician into numerous sections, looking at it from a patient's needs point of view. I discuss the merits of occasionally paternalistic approaches (telling the patient what to do) but the far greater value of advising, informing and guiding short of this. The idea is to start to get the reader to identify his or her limits and to appreciate, even feel good, about them.

A breach of trust

I visited an old lady with one of her periodic infective exacerbations of her chronic obstructive pulmonary disease (COPD) one night. She not only had this disease to contend with but also for some ten years had suffered from a slowly deteriorating chronic lymphocytic leukaemia – as had her son in the same household. Both needed chemotherapy for it.

She was poorly but just this side of being admitted to the hospital, which in any case was closed to emergency admissions at the time. I explained to the two visiting daughters who lived nearby, and who were middle-aged professional people, that Mum should be alright with the treatment, but what to look out for, and call me if needed. They asked about her blood problem and I said her leukaemia was under control presently and did not think it was complicating her chest problem.

The old lady was a retired teacher and could be quite fierce. We got on well though, but she told me off very firmly the next time I saw her because the nature of her blood disorder, the leukaemia, had been a secret. Even though the daughters knew she had something wrong they had been given no label for it; now they knew their brother's problem too. The chemotherapy, the visits to hospital, on one occasion a blood transfusion, had all been kept from the daughters and I had breached this confidence.

The following year she got generally worse and suffered much, from her chest, in the last stages of her life. She did say she was pleased in the end that all her family knew what was going on with her and therefore her son, which was her way of forgiving me for breaking the conspiracy, though sometimes I suspect she did not really mean it.

References

1. Illich I. *Limits to Medicine: medical nemesis – the expropriation of health* London: Marion Boyars, 2001.

2. Gothill M. What do doctors want? Altruism and satisfaction in general practice *Family Practice* 1998; **15**: S36–9.

3. Elwyn G. Idealistic, impractical, impossible? Shared decision making in the real world *British Journal of General Practice* 2006; **56**: 403–4 [editorial].

4. Deale A, Chalder T, Wessely S. Illness beliefs and treatment outcome in chronic fatigue syndrome *Journal of Psychosomatic Research* 1998; **45**: 77–83.

5. Bennet G. The doctor's losses: ideals versus realities *British Medical Journal* 1998; **316**: 1238–40.

CHAPTER 4

Medical status and the expectations this creates

The position of doctors and GPs in particular in society affects our self-perception and
level of confidence. This chapter discusses the frailty of medical status and the conflicts
it creates within ourselves. Status for a competitive group like GPs is also about our
standing in the medical community. In coping with the myriad uncertainties of our job
we need to understand our own drives and the regard in which we are held, in general,
by our patients. From there we can start to negotiate a realistic path with them.

Status arises from a complexity of factors. Is it the same concept as respect? One
tends to give a certain greater respect to the man with the gun, at least as long as
he is a danger to us. The teacher who delivers a smooth, clear and inspiring talk
gains our respect, but the status of those in the education service is stubbornly
below, for instance, our own. Politicians are routinely awarded little respect, however, yet the Prime Minister clearly has status. Doctors seem to thrive on a degree
of both, so they can remain contented, although most find it easier to admit to a
wish for respect rather than a higher rank in society. So it is worth exploring status and respect in some detail, because an understanding of this helps our confidence and effectiveness. Deconstructing our ideas about status can help us to be
clearer and more honest with ourselves, at the risk of being provocative.

Some years ago I was approached by a careers fair organiser and asked to speak to
some sixth formers, who were contemplating university entrance, about becoming a
doctor. It didn't go well, or at least it went differently from expected.

The teacher chairing the meeting had wanted a dreary run-through of the passage
through medical school including how to get in – far too short term a goal. I took
the view that any 16-year-old who doesn't have the initiative to get these facts is
unlikely to thrive as a medic. They can quickly round up all the information they
need and set about lining up appropriate CVs complete with declarations of a
love of science and a deep caring for others, demonstrated by brief spasms of voluntary work, a fortnight's work experience in the NHS and a string of A's. They
can do all that and they can get into medical school, but have they figured out
whether they will enjoy it and whether they will be content? For self-content-
ment is deeply linked to status and it is disingenuous to pretend that no such

shards of selfishness exist. Would the clamour for medical school places exist if the status awarded by society to doctors were to be reduced to that of, for instance, the supermarket shelf-stacker?

I had discussed money, TV doctors, rank and authority, ambition, aspirations, patients (and the varied attitude doctors have towards them) and the pleasures of intellectual growth. She had expected a sales job, for I am a known enthusiast for medicine and relish the work I do, but my sales technique was a bit subtle. Illustrating the rewards of the job by quoting multiples of a teacher's salary was, I admit, tactless. I took it upon myself to point out that some clinical work is intellectually mundane – not just in primary care by any means – so the brilliant mind hungry for new stimulation might be unhappy, as in many jobs, and has to find other ways of feeding itself. Doctors are generally competitive and ambitious, and yet liable to find ourselves at 40 or so in permanent jobs, often a little short of the starring role of which we had dreamt, though not as dissatisfied as might appear from the medical press.[1] The status we seek and will get is high, as seen by patients, but our peer group by this age consists of other experienced senior doctors, largely therefore of equals, so we might feel we have not achieved so much. We should think this through. And the doctor who comes to terms with this plateau will be more contented and, to boot, more effective.

So talking of the privileges and responsibilities of medical status seemed a reasonable angle; it is not pure altruism that drives us. The result was that I was given only some faltering thanks by a flabbergasted teacher who struggled out the sentiment that I had presented one of the most candid talks she had heard in recent years. No doubt she filled in a suitable evaluation form to the main organiser and this explains why, to my dismay, that to date no further invitation from this outfit has dropped on to my doormat.

Fabulous doctors

There can be no higher status for doctors than those who are part of the crew on the spaceship USS *Enterprise*, in the science fiction programme *Star Trek*.

For over 20 years each series has featured a core cast of the captain, first officer, doctor and a couple of other senior officers who have various adventures. The ranking given the doctor would seem to be third or fourth in command of a huge ship, a position the Royal Navy would I assume find rather uncomfortable on the bridge of the *Ark Royal*.

The doctor is of course very clever and technically brilliant, but sometimes emotional and therefore not as perfect as the captain. The plot lines frequently rely on some previously unheard of medical crisis for which a physical solution is found in the nick of time. It has to be said the plot lines are often complex, presenting ethical and philosophical dilemmas as much as straight action hero stuff.

This image of a genius problem solver seems more in keeping with the US model of medicine, in which the body is seen in technical terms. Ever more ingenious technical, chemical or sometimes psychological solutions are sought and sometimes found to counter human malfunctions. Proud as one is to be in the same profession as these heroes, there is a discomfort that expectations are sky high and that, so long as the lay public are led to think that if only they can find a doctor clever enough that their problems are solvable, then we are doomed to disappoint.

Where does this high status of doctors come from? It was certainly not always present, and nineteenth-century literature, like *Punch* magazine, was only too happy to finger the self-interested doctors and useless remedies they peddled. And Florence Nightingale's vocation, of course in many ways more effective than doctors, was to be deprecated at the time. But through careful grooming and regulating of the professions in the last century, first doctors then nurses have become admired pillars of society with respect and status. Perhaps we live in an age that likes to flatten the rise of even well-proven reputations but doctors and health staff remain high on any journalist's compilation of those whom the public trust most.[2] The journalists, of course, are barely on the list at all.

The media hero medic is a major hazard to real-life doctors and patients. Not only does the wonderful doctor on TV show commitment, knowledge and skill, so raising the patient's expectations, but also leaves the medical part of the audience feeling inadequate and pathetic. In real life we are unable to be even remotely accurate in the prediction of death in an individual case, whereas the patient in the soap opera is awarded his or her suspended sentence with lethal accuracy. How feeble then, in our world, not to be able say whether a patient will be fit enough for a holiday next Easter, now they know he or she has heart disease or cancer. And how useless it feels when, if it is accepted we cannot avert the catastrophic illness, we can't even help with holiday plans.

A clever exercise in group learning to facilitate individuals seeing where they might be placed within a team, and what role they might adopt in which they are comfortable, confident and valued by the group, goes like this.

The team is set the task of choosing the half dozen most useful survivors on a desert island shipwreck. They have a list of perhaps 15 people with different skills and backgrounds, and the group has to choose which six of these might be able to become a self-supporting team and thereby survive. The rest get killed off in the fictional shipwreck. The 15 includes difficult choices like a baby, an uneducated farm labourer, an agoraphobic cook, whatever – and includes an elderly doctor.

The educational process works unexpectedly, because it does not matter who the group chooses, merely how they set about the grisly task. People get passionate, or rebellious, or opt out and sit in a corner. Some within the group will listen better than others, while some will be keen for consensus decisions and others want to win by force of argument and majority vote. The learning for the group is in the reflection afterwards, ideally via video, of how they acted as individuals tackling the task, and how this might be done better, more effectively and more in a team spirit. Naturally the idea is for the group to carry these insights as individuals into their own working teams or partnerships, and environment.

However, one person the group will reliably place amongst the survivors will be the medic. Like in a balloon debate at school,* where if there is a doctor on board he or she has a massively unfair advantage and much enhanced survival chance, the conventional view of the doctor is as an indispensable person. Even though the perils of heat, cold, thirst and starvation are far more likely in our shipwreck scenario than serious diseases treatable with local materials, the doctor is voted on to the survivor list. A politician, who might have leadership qualities, and an artist, who might have useful practical know-how, tend not to make it.

That we are given this great status is apparent, then, though the reasoning behind it is complicated. Status in a society is not of course something a committee ponders on and then awards after due diligence and logic; it has a large emotive component. The clinical professions themselves work hard to keep it, promoting themselves politically and in the media as well as materially. The areas that we might look at to understand our status and then decide if we deserve it are in our values. These can be professional, intellectual and materialistic amongst others.

Having pigeon-holed present entrants to the healing professions, a comparison between our own motives at that age and now might prove to be a further uncomfortable and perhaps even brutal reality.

After all there is a tension between our desire for 'professionalism' and our baser drives that needs acknowledging. Professionalism is a clumsy word but encompasses most of the good stuff we would like to think we do. Tenets like doing no deliberate harm, placing patients invariably first and our own needs (like getting home) second, and treating all the varied specimens of humanity we encounter with equal respect, are absolute essentials for being trusted. Of equal importance and value is the knowledge of one's limitations, communicating with colleagues and keeping up to date – under all circumstances. A characteristic of the burden of being professional is that it is self-driven and regulated, of course (though, just in case the system fails, it is now considered a professional duty to report on the significant failings of one's colleagues). There is a large body of literature discussing professional values and a large and expensive body of the profession itself to pronounce and regulate them.

Yet sometimes our professional values are less a source of pride and support, and more of a problem. In the face of the demands of home for our time, plodding on until the last patient has been thoroughly sorted out, the last journal read and last letter signed it can sometimes feel almost too much (though we manage somehow).

The simple supermarket shelf-stacker has an easier task, does he not?

---

* The premise behind a balloon debate is that there are several individuals in a hot-air balloon that is too heavy and, for any to survive the plummet to earth, all bar one has to be jettisoned. The individuals represent professions, like a social worker or orchestra conductor, and the class hears their case, then debates and votes on their value.

Food

Idealism during the penultimate medical school year was strong, and still is, though I like to think that some pragmatism has been learned. Over one particular huge carbohydrate loading session, generally termed lunch, with one of the housemen on the surgical firm to which I was attached, he said that it is more important to eat than to attend to a patient in pain. I was amazed at the callousness. His rationale was that you did not know when you would next get a chance to eat.

My resolve to ignore the advice lasted until my second week or so of the house year when the inhumanity of the hours was getting at me and the patient in pain was becoming a repeated challenge. There are circumstances in which abandoning the starchy dollop of a hospital canteen lunch was warranted, but they were rare.

Is this unprofessional? No, because on arriving at the patient's bedside I can more efficiently deal with the problem if my stomach is settled. And I can see more patients later on too. This first conflict of idealistic professional values and real life, when I had to give myself permission to be human, was an introduction to the painful discrepancy between what wonderful doctors are expected to do, and what they can.

Does our shelf-stacker use professional values to go by? Well, one can assume he or she aims to do no harm. Opportunities for the GP to do harm abound, certainly, but so too can a careless or untrained shelf-stacker create hazardous towers of goods, risking showers of beans tins or smashed bottles of cheap, pungent wine. The culture of working to defined hours is inherent to such jobs, which might imply that the shelf-stacker's priority is more self-interested than selfless. But the realistic shelf-stacker knows that he or she simply cannot finish every shelf in the shop in one shift, but must let someone know where he or she got to before finishing. Let us remember that, after the decades of frustration and exploitation by the system, leaving at the moment the pay stops is now common amongst the shift-working medical classes. Most modern supermarkets have customer relations training so the dutiful shelf-stacker, when approached by the shopper, can at least pretend to be respectful and helpful no matter what he or she feels about the shopper's value to society (and even if the customer is recognised as the doctor he or she doesn't like). And most shops will treat a sale as confidential unless it becomes a police matter, as anyone trying to trace the origin of flowers on Valentine's Day will discover.

But why would a shelf-stacker be bothered to do a good job? There must be positive and negative reasons. Taking pride in the job and pleasure in pleasing others (like the manager and the customers) is hardly a universal human trait, but it is common. It is not the exclusive preserve of the caring professions. Perhaps in this instance there is the aesthetic pleasure of setting rows of cereal packets in an inviting, attractive line. There is certainly some science in selling and the length of shelf awarded to a particular product is a careful economic calculation. The manager might wish to make all these decisions, but he or she is unwise to ignore the stacker entirely and might well have started from that role at one point. Naturally our stacker is also afraid of the manager, and part of the reason for stacking shelves well is therefore the stick rather than the carrot, but no manager who used the stick approach alone ever managed to nurture loyal staff who would stay behind a bit on December 24th.

To make a comparison between the professional values of doctors and those of an unskilled manual worker might feel cheap or unreasonable. That the GP's overall purpose is on a higher plane than our manual worker friend is true after all. The point is that the shelf-stacker looks up to the doctor but not especially because the latter has a set of admirable and august professional values unknown amongst the lower classes. They can spot a lazy doctor and are no more forgiving of that, or surprised by it, than we are on encountering a lazy checkout operator.

We are differentiated by exam success though. The criteria for entry to medical school is high – a row of A's at A level and an articulate, carefully crafted personal statement plus preparation for competitive structured interview selection, are each mandatory. Entering medical school is then a shock to the majority of students who find on arrival at university, for the first time, that they are not top of the class. Or that they cannot get to be top without extreme effort. All medical school teachers hate the look on the good students' faces on getting B's, and C's, only a few ever getting the coveted but hitherto relatively easy A for any given piece of work. Prior to this most were bright sixth formers finding only moderate challenge in the content of their A level courses and, by applying some effort and focus, achieved their ambitions. By definition these students have learned to work effectively but most have an inner awareness in the sixth form that they are naturally good, and, when this is combined with the necessary effort, they can easily be at the top. But at medical school they meet the cream of all the other schools and the new peer group provides a jolt; much of the rest of their medical school class seems seriously bright or at least good at appearing so.

The competitive instinct is there, though, not even below the surface, and might either boost their confidence or destroy it. Of course medical school is a continuous run of examinations, assessments and tests, so opportunities to do well are frequent. Yet the reassurance the student now seeks by being good at tests does not automatically translate into clinical self-confidence. Many a nervous student, measurably excellent in both exams and skills like history taking, remains anxious that he or she cannot cope. He or she has glimpsed at the vast confidence-sapping volume of knowledge within medicine, and no one has told him or her how to decide what he or she needs to know. To date it was quite realistic to 'know' the A level chemistry syllabus, or even the latest thinking and research in some remote field of cell biology. It could be written down, visualised. But the concept of an unlimited syllabus is inconceivable, and like the so-called imaginary numbers in mathematics (which form the square roots of negative integers) cannot easily be pictured. The temptation to just try to learn as much as possible is then strong, even in the face of rationality, and because these students are capable of learning a lot, and driven by each other, many do just that. Then on entry to general practice training the 'syllabus' becomes encyclopaedic at least at first sight, and many registrars flounder in the torrent of their own expectations.

Knowing a great deal is impressive, in the same way that a teacher who can quote massive tracts of Shakespeare or a politician who has a formidable grasp of statistical detail to brow-beat an opponent with his or her case is impressive. We can debate usefulness elsewhere. The truth is that the combination of the types of personality who enter medical school and the impossibility of 'knowing' medicine does not stop some from trying. We might think that the resulting bulging memory banks possessed by such GPs are much respected, and they are great for peer group point scoring, but they do not confer great status and confidence, and do not necessarily lead to sounder decision making. This knowledge is broad at least as much as deep. The vastness of the territory, which doctors have to know especially for their hideous exams, is such that they have to assimilate a great deal at high speed. For the most part this impresses our peers as clinicians, rather than patients. The amount of knowledge needed to advise any one individual patient might not appear to them to be huge, though it might well tot up on repeated encounters. At the risk of repetition, patients value the doctor's manner, time, examination skills and judgement before neat braininess, which comes over as rather scary. We are not necessarily accurate at assessing our own knowledge level and subsequent educational needs either.[3] However, the temptation to try to impress patients with braininess is strong, and achieved at least subconsciously by the use of complex language. Baffling patients with science is an art in itself, perhaps fortunately a dying one. The more educated assertive patients, insensitive to the demands on the clinician's time, will not let jargon get in the way and if they cannot get a clearer version will threaten to use the internet, 'alternative practitioners' or even the Sunday papers for accessible wisdom. On the other hand, this perceived general erudition of clinicians does sometimes lead to misunderstandings about what we can and cannot pronounce on. Many GPs have had requests for information and guidance on marital law, housing policy, debt counselling or educational provision come up in the course of their consultations. This might be superficially amusing but might well reflect an issue having a major impact on the patient's health. The confident GP defers to a superior authority on this – if in doubt, try the Citizens Advice Bureau – because they know it is better to look vulnerable now than foolish later. It reflects that we would be worldly enough to be able to discover something, even a legal issue, fairly easily, whereas our patient might not know where to start. That so many patients face apparent injustice affecting their health is perhaps a political issue rather than a medical one, but that we are approachable as a trusted, sensible and competent friend is a compliment that should make us feel good. The danger with wandering beyond our expertise is that experience tells us the patient might have not told us the whole story, omitting details that might have made us less sympathetic to their plight.

Useful knowledge

It is easy to snipe, but for most of us which of the following has proven crucial, or is likely to, in our working lives? Knowing how to:

- manage polyarteritis nodosa
- fix a car's damp distributor
- mediate between squabbling colleagues
- write a legal report
- prioritise an agenda
- use a computerised database

- navigate around a new hospital

- clean up a vomiting toddler

- give CPR

- give a talk to a lay audience?

And which of these was taught as part of your basic training? The chances are polyarteritis was in there somewhere. Yet fewer than 1 in 50 doctors, and many fewer nurses, is actually involved in a case.

To draw up a 'syllabus' might actually be easier than one thinks to equip the learner with most of the knowledge and skills he or she will need, but it might well look intellectually dull, and therefore unworthy.

The image of Harley Street is fascinating. Rooms there are for rent, by anyone, though at a rent that makes it more sensible to consider paying hourly rather than monthly. The eminent doctors of the capital displaying awesome qualifications are lined up, every possible speciality and sub-speciality being available. Fees are vast as are, of course, expenses. But amongst the brilliant and cerebral top doctors are the average and very occasionally the venal, charging similarly vast fees. Undercover journalists cut their teeth exposing these rogues, yet the dominance of the address as the prime medical site of the nation goes unchallenged.

There are many fair reasons for consulting a doctor privately, like speed, convenience, time and atmosphere, especially when someone else like an insurance company is paying. What is perennially sad is that many patients also believe, against objective evidence and the ethics of 90 per cent of specialists, that a paid-for opinion is a better one. That by going to ever 'cleverer' and more expensive doctors eventually someone will be able to cure the incurable, and give good news for once. The most extreme examples of this are those heart-rending cases publicised from time to time of dying children or young adults who are raising money as often as not to go to abroad. The nothing-to-lose approach to high-tech surgery raises hopes, and the fees, generally into six figures, raise them further. No greater cry can there be than 'give the money or my child will die'. The case of Child B in Cambridge,* who had a rare leukaemia, was one such in which a child whose disorder had relapsed, was denied treatment by the NHS not for reasons of economy as initially implied, but because there was no treatment of any use. Eventually a benefactor paid up for the controversial experimental therapy that the family had asked for, sadly to no avail. A courageous chief executive in the local NHS was prepared to back the decision publicly, a chill rationality against the emotive pleas of but-you-must-do-something.

The point of this is that the actual height of the fees – in Child B's case, some £75,000 – adds status to the clinician in the same way as we are more in awe of a lawyer who charges a thousand a day than one who scrapes by on a third of that. But we GPs know really that the fees do not reflect ability, just location, field, and perhaps glamour.

---

* See Chapter 11 for further details of this case.

More mundanely, in the average town, the great majority of doctors have no significant private practice or even, perhaps, a wish for one. Their income comes from the NHS with some small peripheral extras perhaps. Comparisons can be overvalued yet we must remember that the median income in our average town in 2003 – the point at which half the population earns more and half less – is about £22,000 p.a. This is more useful than mean income, which is distorted by extremes, especially at the top end. So the senior clinicians locally, GPs and consultants, will get four to five times the median from their NHS work (and the senior nurse around double). This will allow them to live in visible comfort if not ostentation.

47

Bigger houses, bigger Mercedes, exclusive schooling, and the outward trappings of wealth must contribute to the status clinicians have in their society, including our average town. The fact that in many walks of life status brings contacts and opportunity for more wealth and thus more status is an accepted part of the system; nothing succeeds like success. Doctors might not have the business chances and mind of an entrepreneur, but they still choose the private golf course over the municipal one.

So we have considered our professional values and, whilst we are viewed as more personally honest than Joe Bloggs, otherwise we are not that exceptional. The status gained from sheer brain power is a help, used by doctors unsure of their position and role to keep their knowledge to themselves in the face of increasingly rebellious patients. But others whose job is regarded as needing a good brain, like teachers or engineers or lawyers, do not enjoy quite the status of the clinician so there must be more. Then there is the simple worship of wealth, our own and that of others, and the deference given to those with it, and certainly even GPs gain respect from the simple fact of being well-off. However, we still have an unease or nervousness about ourselves that suggests there is more to this.

Dedication to the job can take many forms. We pay carers in residential homes the minimum wage to spend nights, for example, wiping bottoms. The briefest of reflection makes one wonder whether this is dedication or desperation. The opportunities for any work for many of these carers are few, in that they might be trapped with no qualifications and no child care arrangements, and so they take whatever work can fit into the hours the kids are looked after by the family. But it is not just desperation; there is real visible care there too (with, as usual, notable if rare exceptions). Does society award them higher status than say an equivalently paid factory worker?

Some of the esteem in which GPs are held might be thought to arise from the more disgusting sides to the job we do. Splashing around in the various fluids of which the human body is capable of exuding or poking fingers into unspeakable orifices is everyday stuff for many of us. Certainly the level of tolerance of the repellent that is needed is too high for many people to consider doing our work – 'Oh God, I couldn't do that!' our friends cry. But this in itself does not grant GPs particular status. Nor for that matter does the grim work of the forensic pathologist or the casualty nurse, or the regular day of the proctologist and the incontinence adviser give them special credit, merely admiration. And rather more than the care worker, who has the same olfactory challenge. All that has happened with all us care workers is that we have become detached and unaffected by this side of the work we do, because we know we could not cope if we kept feeling repelled, and we know the patient needs us to be caring. Society seems at one level to understand that some people can learn to cope with the fouler side of human life, but prefers not to think about it too much and so awards little status for this ability.

Similarly the patients with whom we deal vary in their level of vulnerability and attractiveness. Here the hypocrisy of status is rife. The doctor who numbers amongst his or her patients the great and the good seems to carry a higher regard than the one who battles on with the derelict and the drugged. A case might easily be made that the care and management of a patient with learning difficulties and in considerable poverty is a tougher challenge than the same health issue in a patient of means and resource. Each needs a similar level of clinical knowledge and ability, but the former might require much greater communication skills and psycho-social knowledge. Yet the social status of the patient rubs on to the GP or other doctor. Exceptions abound, and amongst ourselves rather than the chattering classes this difference might be smaller. But the consequence is that recruiting to a post looking after the middle and upper classes is easier than to a job involving striving with lower strata.

The media image of the nurse and doctor is not inaccurate in the hours we do. Here the cliché has truth, of the sacrificed weekends and punctuated social life.* Long hours are engrained in the culture of the hospital doctors now in middle age, from their misspent youth doing shattering one-in-threes. It has taken the bureaucrats of Brussels to fight their corner for decent working hours for junior doctors, and they still remain longer than average workers. In the meantime we all experience patients being sympathetic about long hours: asking after our welfare, admiring our stamina. These moments of appreciation are no substitute for a decent but illusive lunch break, but do make one aware of the public view.

Power, as any GCSE student of physics can tell us, is a function of time and energy. If energy equates to a doctor's activity and time is measured in units of a day, say, then the busy clinician who does a lot in his or her day, usually by making the working part of it long, might be seen to have more power and thus status. Activity includes not just seeing patients but attendance at meetings and, from their colleagues' point of view, a continuous visible presence at the workplace. More hours spent there mean more is done in our unit of a day.

So are we guilty of working long hours to keep our status? What an appalling thought! But if we feel inadequate, and not in control, then the least we can do is be around in case we are useful. We are vulnerable to checking behaviour (see Chapter 6) and the secondary benefit is an appreciation of how dedicated we must be. After all, a wealth of research on the different speeds at which doctors in particular work, whilst open to charges of being flawed and being politically motivated, tends to conclude that faster doctors are not necessarily worse.[4]

---

* The dropping of on-call and its replacement by voluntary paid shifts has had the unplanned consequence of the loss of a water-tight reason for skipping an unwanted or tedious social obligation – 'I'm sorry, on call'.

Status within the caring professions

The ranking amongst the medical profession goes back a long way. Before 1800 there was no doubt that the physicians, who had a royal college and had trained for five years at university, were the leaders of the profession. They made a living amongst their social equals and the aristocracy – the carriage trade.

The poor, of course, had no access to such grand people and made use of whatever quackery was available. Apothecaries emerged in the eighteenth century, initially dispensing but soon prescribing and advising as well. In 1800 the former Company of Surgeons, descendants of the heroic military surgeons and barbers of the Middle Ages, became the Royal College of Surgeons. Apothecaries began to evolve into those who were surgeon-apothecaries, those becoming physician-apothecaries, as well as those who were concentrating on the retail trade and dispensing. The surgeon-apothecaries became the first 'general practitioners', over the next 50 years or so, but the Apothecaries Act in 1815 clearly obliged them to dispense on the instruction of a physician, thereby establishing their rank position. This act started to regulate the education of apothecaries and doctors, and in 1858 the General Medical Council was created and charged with licensing education and standards. The physicians and surgeons had their own exams but a GP could practise if a licentiate of the Royal College of Physicians and a member of the Royal College of Surgeons. That said, surgeon-chemists continued to the end of the nineteenth century, often relying more on the retail trade in shampoo and toothbrushes than their income from operating. As such their status was fairly lowly, thriving as they did with the GPs amongst the lower classes.

GPs from the start of the Friendly Societies in the later nineteenth century, and then the Lloyd George Act of 1911, began to get income from capitation fees paid by the government or an organisation for looking after working men no matter what their state of health. In some schemes the family as well as the breadwinner might have been covered too. As they had little to offer in terms of biological effectiveness they were saved from those embarrassments of failure that a fee-for-service system might be thought to generate. Arguably they had little incentive to intervene where intervention was pointless too, though as compassionate and knowledgeable people they were valued in a crisis. What did tend to happen, with a registered population, was that the GP was more rooted in the community than the physician or hospital surgeon. Many would have had a low income, similar to their patients, although by the time of the start of the NHS most GPs had 'mixed' lists of wealthy and poor, and used a sliding scale of charges to reflect this. Young doctors would nevertheless have to carve a reputation by practising effectively amongst the poorer classes before the wealthier would risk attending them, and if they had a consultancy at the hospital their prestige, and fees, duly rose.

Huge advances in surgery in the inter-war and war years brought greater regard for the surgeons, who from the start of the NHS were, like the physicians, now seen as specialists who dealt entirely within their field. The need for a specialist to have a general practice disappeared and they concentrated on the work in hospital.

This potted (and inadequate) history is to remind us of the roots of medical hierarchy, which remain today. Status amongst doctors is little studied. There is a ranking by branch of profession, so the senior thoracic or general surgeon is seen up there at the top, with the cardiologist and neurologist. Background is the first feature to be factored in to the status sum – where they trained both for their first degree and subsequently. This is both by country and university, preference being given rather obviously to attendance at the ancient universities of the UK without much objective evidence of superiority where it matters. Sheer length of service then adds status, but in the end the profession still has its major and minor branches, the latter conferring lower status. Ear, nose and throat (ENT) surgery does not hold the power of neurosurgery, and the geriatrician is less highly ranked than the intensive therapy unit (ITU) consultant. GPs have always felt themselves to be junior to the specialists, possibly because for most of our history this branch of the profession has taken those doctors who have not made it in hospital (an exception was the 1980s when primary care was seen as far more worthwhile than most jobs, and training places were heavily competed for, and since 2006 we have seen another resurgence in the popularity of general practice). GPs have their ranking system too, with involvement in academia, politics or education perhaps conferring an advantage. Location confuses the matter further, so an inner-city non-teaching hospital consultant post is of lower status than the charms of a major London teaching hospital. These desirability factors then become self-perpetuating, in that the most admired candidates of any one generation go for and get the higher-status jobs, so the posts around them become more attractive by association. This is the 'critical mass' effect in which a thriving and respected department with most posts filled will always recruit to its occasional vacancies more easily than the corresponding area in a neighbouring trust that has a lot of vacancies. Finally, to add to background, length of service, the job factor and the location factor, there are of course factors that individual doctors bring so that their reputation and status is moved either up or down, to some extent by merit or demerit.

Proof that status is linked to the job is seen by the way consultants are given 'merit awards'. These secretive payments are enhancements, sometimes large, to salary, which are decided on by small local committees. That the disgraced paediatric heart surgeons of Bristol all held high awards shows how the job rather than the individual is rewarded!

Why should the heart surgeon be so regarded? A characteristic of the higher-status medics is toughness, perhaps. They have usually worked hard even for a hard-working profession, and passed exams in their spare time. They will have some research work under their belt – but so do most consultants. The nature of their job is dramatic; you can't get much more dramatic than opening up a heart. To most of us this will require an admirable cool. The physician impresses, as above, with a vast knowledge and understanding, one hopes, of the unusual and complex case. 'The mind of the physician' wrote Richard Asher, that doyen of the Middlesex Hospital 'and that structure which corresponds to the mind of the surgeon' demonstrates this snobbery.

Nurses' ranking in the eyes of society is interestingly complex. An ICM survey in 2001 showed across all groups nurses were viewed as having a status – for which read respect, perhaps – second to doctors but ahead of teachers, lawyers, bankers, architects, computer consultants and management consultants. They are, more predictably, ahead of politicians and journalists, who of course vie to provide the baseline; the nurses scored 7.65 on ICM's score out of 10, against 8.23 for the doctors (and 5.04 for the hacks).[5] On an absolute level nurses might be quite pleased by the result, which no doubt is cited, or at least alluded to, in pay talks.

The gap in status awarded to the two professions is not that big, which might be a surprise to those doctors who remain fond of the current hierarchy. Discussion in the primary care press in the last few years has been about delegating the care of more patients from doctors to nurses but the Royal College of General Practitioners said that, whilst 40 per cent of patients can be nurse managed, you only know that in retrospect at the end of a consultation. The feeling is that 40 per cent of the patients at presentation could not be identified and seen by nurses safely. In fact the evidence is that patients requesting acute care can decide themselves by whom they are seen and get it right most of the time; they are happy with nurse care, not least because the nurse consulting style is less hurried and perceived as more listening. Outcomes such as investigations, referrals, prescriptions and follow-ups show little difference between doctor and nurse consultations in acute primary care for this group of patients.[6] This is therefore in keeping with the ICM's survey information rather than doctors' views. However, a caveat has to be that the threshold of taking responsibility of care, whereby patients seek help, has certainly fallen during the 1990s and so a number of patients who 20 years ago were not contacting the NHS at all, but were in fact coping alone, are now using the NHS. Many of these 'low threshold' cases will have come into this category of acute primary care, but also the corresponding threshold of referral into secondary care has changed. We send in all the suspicious chest pains now, and quite right too. Much of both of the low-threshold groups will have been happily nurse managed. The comparator is thus not strictly GP/nurse management but nurse/patient management.

Given that one might argue that nurses are quite a bit less academic on entry into training, have half the training length of doctors, are far more restricted in their treatment options, and are rarely in a situation of final responsibility, then the status awarded by the population to them warrants explanation. We competitive doctors are prone to feeling threatened by this. Of course the above parameters are not the only important values in the patient's eyes; they value such skills as approachability, safety, time, and an understanding of the state of being ill, which perhaps doctors underestimate. Possibly whilst the medical profession and indeed this book advocate greater patient empowerment and responsibility, there is a part of the patient that likes the paternalism of many a kindly nurse saying what should be done, on a homely level, rather than the GP sharing options too liberally. Even Shakespeare put the nurse in that role in *Romeo and Juliet* when the nurse was initially the jolly friend of Juliet, although later changing her view and exhorting her to follow her parents', rather than her heart's, desire (for the record, Juliet nevertheless chose not to take that option).[7]

Perhaps the truth is less clear cut and patients do not differentiate between doctors and nurses as much as the professions think. They just like the thought that we are there when needed.

It gets worse. The medical raconteur Rob Buckman describes how he was first on the scene at a car accident where the patient was injured and bleeding on the pavement, surrounded by incompetent bystanders.[8] At the time he was a second-year medical student and naturally he felt able to take charge. Just as the responsibilities he had taken upon himself dawned on his panicking brain, rescue came from the rear of the crowd. As the group split, a sensible and concerned looking chap emerged, shouting to the gawping bystanders to let him through. 'I'm a social worker' he explained, and the crowd sighed with relief.

The general public puts all of us care workers in the same category, on roughly the same overcrowded pedestal.

Conclusion

It is reasonable and understandable to seek status. But it is important for the confident clinician to understand the irrationality of status within society and within our professions, and to seek contentment when by dint of personality he or she fails to please his or her inner drive. We cannot avoid being influenced by society's odd values but we can be a touch disdainful.

References

1.   Goldacre M, Lambert TW, Parkhouse J. The views of doctors in the UK about their own professional position and the NHS reforms *Journal of Public Health Medicine* 1998; **20**: 86–92.

2.   Ipsos MORI poll, November 2006.

3.   Tracey J, Arroll B, Barham P, *et al*. The validity of GPs' self assessment of knowledge *British Medical Journal* 1997; **315**: 1426–8.

4.   Black A. Reconfiguring health systems *British Medical Journal* 2002; **325**: 1290–3.

5.   ICM poll for the Institute of Public Policy Research, September 2001.

6.   Laurent M, Reeves D, Hermens R, *et al*. The substitution of doctors by nurses in primary care (review) *Cochrane Database of Systemic Reviews* 2005, Cd001271.

7.   Shakespeare W. *Romeo and Juliet*, act III, scene v.

8.   Buckman R. *Out of Practice* London: Billing & Son, 1978.

CHAPTER 5

The few certainties of life

There are some certainties in medical care, and some cases where traditionally a small uncertainty is expressed but which is actually so small as to be truly and literally negligible. Then there are some consultations where there are genuinely two or more viable and reasonable decision paths available, and the GP should go to some lengths to get the patient to choose between them. This chapter also starts to cover the deficiencies of evidence-based medicine in a typical clinical scenario, and some pitfalls for unwary GPs whose uncertainties are proving difficult to handle.

Although there are circumstances when NHS accountants might welcome this flexibility, it is, on the whole, alarming to hear that $2 + 2$ does not always equal 4.

Bertrand Russell, the eminent twentieth-century mathematician and philosopher, when confronted by someone who thought that $2 + 2$ always equalled 4, remarked

> You are quite right except in marginal cases – and it is only in marginal cases that you are doubtful whether a certain animal is a dog or a certain length is less than a metre. Two must be two of something and the proposition '2 and 2 are 4' is useless unless it can be applied. Two dogs and two dogs are certainly four dogs, but cases arise in which you are doubtful whether two of them are dogs. 'Well at any rate, there are four animals' you may say. But there are micro organisms concerning which it is doubtful whether they are animals or plants. 'Well, then living organisms' you say. But there are things of which it is doubtful whether they are living organisms or not. You will be driven into saying 'Two entities and two entities are four entities'. When you have told me what you mean by entities, we will resume the argument.

This uncertainty really does not help in the average, hurried, NHS consultation. If something as obviously certain as the addition of two integers can, by the sophistry of pedantic academics, be made to feel if not uncertain, then definitely not guaranteed, then how do we know anything? Naturally it might be interesting as an exercise, the next time a patient asks for a guarantee, to discuss the philosophical basis for his or her request, and to prove that it cannot be met. However, it is likely that the clinician who proves to a patient that absolute certainty cannot be attained will him or herself be labelled impossible. A label, of course, that might or might not be justified.

This tension between the human need to know what is going on and the cover-all-possibilities school of reassurance has to be understood by the GP at some depth, because a patient in an anxious state is reluctant to accept it. And, actually, the patient might well be right.

It is important to know what a proof is, not least because it is a thing of rare beauty. We need to stick with maths here, even having shown the philosophical wobbliness of what might have seemed a basic precept.

The ancient Chinese knew that the square of the hypotenuse is the sum of the squares of the other two sides in a right-angled triangle, because they had noticed it. No matter how many triangles they tried it on, the formula, crucial to the construction of buildings and impressive engineering feats from ancient dynasties, worked. But they never actually proved it could be so for any and all sizes of right-angled triangle, although they were sure it was. Sure enough, in fact to trust the formula in their calculations. The Greeks, meanwhile, got on and proved it.[*]

Mathematicians have striven ever since to develop proofs of their theorems that display elegance and vigour, and of course ever more baffling complexity. Everyone else, perhaps especially life scientists, has to accept something less.

Pythagoras' theorem

Figure 5.1: Pythagoras' theorem

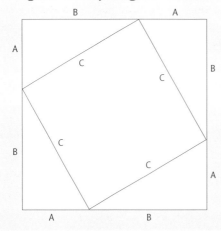

The area in the middle square may be calculated as the area of the outer square – $(a + b)^2$ – less the area in the four triangles, each of which is $1/2 \times a \times b$.

So we get
$(a + b)^2 - 4 \times 1/2 ab$
i.e. $a^2 + b^2 + ab + ba - 2ab$
$= a^2 + b^2$

But the centre square is also $c \times c = c^2$

So $a^2 + b^2 = c^2$ for any values of a right-angled triangle

We might be more than reasonably certain that the sun will rise tomorrow morning, or more exactly the earth will continue to rotate relative to the sun for at least the next 24 hours, although we can only guess if we will be around to see it. The fact that the sun has come over the horizon for each day for billions of years makes us feel pretty confident it will do it again. But, on the other hand, we know that the history of the cosmos does include rare calamities such as stars exploding – and so a failure of the dawn tomorrow is slightly more likely than

---

[*] Yet the Parthenon, curiously, has no exact straight lines or right angles, merely very gentle curves giving the illusion of precise horizontal and vertical edges. Pericles' understanding of geometry was more sophisticated still.

someone finding a triangle for which Pythagoras got it wrong. Yet the billions to one chance of the earth not surviving the next 24 hours is sufficiently remote for us not to worry about it. Therefore there must be a point somewhere, short of the point of absolute proof but close to it, at which the gap between them is unimportant in real life. Doctors often have to judge this in order to take the responsibilities their patients demand, but they struggle to do so.

GPs and other clinicians have to learn to look people in the eye and say that

1. Pythagoras was right, and he will still be right tomorrow and, equally truly,

2. the sun will rise in the morning

So there is a point beyond which, although there is technical uncertainty, the room for error and doubt is so small that one can reasonably be certain. Not, it should be noted, 'reasonably certain', but it is reasonable to declare it a certainty.

In clinical medicine a good example is the fluoridation of water. Campaigners against the idea routinely put about graphs and charts for the local politicians to fret over, showing a rise in cancer or some other disease that apparently occurs in association with fluoridation. The public health team can demonstrate that fluoride is dramatically successful at reducing dental caries, and that they can refute the distorted figures of the opposition, whose statistics do not stand up to the most rudimentary examination. But the elected representatives will say to the public health doctors, at whatever committee decides these things, that they believe what they hear from them, but is it not true that an excess of fluoride has been shown to be harmful to bones (fluoridosis)? So how do they know for sure and absolutely that so-called therapeutic amounts are invariably safe? The public health doctor can give reassuring numbers – millions of people, no evidence of harm, long experience, and so on. And the killer question is then, 'Doctor, can you absolutely guarantee that no one will be harmed by this?'

Intellectually, he or she has to say no. An exceedingly rare adverse event is not inconceivable, just by its nature very unlikely. This potential adverse event is so unlikely that it has never been recorded as actually happening – no one has been measurably harmed by fluoridation of water despite thousands of millions of 'doses' drunk. But this observation doesn't technically prove the innocence of the fluoride, and it is within the bounds of imagination, just, that an adverse event would occur. So the doctor says he or she cannot give such an absolute guarantee.

This is the wrong answer, for on this many teeth will rot. The right answer is yes, because the numbers in this sort of case are so close to absolute that we can say the difference is meaningless. (A more sensible way round is to argue the known consequences of not giving the fluoride, with poor dentition and the diseases which follow that, versus the known downsides, which amount to nothing.)

Similarly, the following questions might be, indeed are, asked of GPs and one can answer truthfully in everyday circumstances with a clear yes or no.

▪ Is it safe for my child, who has no known allergies, to have reasonable doses of paracetamol for his pain and/or fever?

▪ Is it safe for me to leave this tiny, unchanging mole with no malignant features?

- Is it better for the baby to sleep on her back?

- Will my cancer get better without treatment?

And many others.

The questions whose answers are above this pragmatic threshold of uncertainty, albeit below a mathematical certainty, are pretty easy and need some knowledge of medicine only. We might call these facts. The next level of questions from patients begins to demand some judgement.

- Is it safe to have this endoscopy?

- Are these antibiotics/antidepressants/antihypertensives etc. safe for me? Or necessary?

- Will you be able to cure me of this early breast/endometrial/skin cancer?

These are situations in which the figures show that the planned happy outcome is highly likely, but it is within many doctors' experience to have encountered an unexpected adverse encounter. We are told that every anaesthetic carries a risk, albeit lower than 1 in 10,000 in optimum circumstances. But consultant anaesthetists will administer far more anaesthetics than this in their professional lifetime and so they cannot honestly guarantee the patient will come round safely from the anaesthetic in all circumstances. Indeed they will probably know of occasional but memorable and entirely unpredicted tragedies. Indeed they might well have been involved in such and carry the emotional scars forever. And the GP knows that the decision to operate began with the (albeit shared) decision to refer.

Media presentations

The measles, mumps and rubella (MMR) vaccine debacle was covered especially during 2001 and 2002, but also currently, by journalists who have a need to make attractive stories. We live in a world of competitive media, and journalists fighting for the public attention have discovered that what sells well is a story in which there are elements of news, mystery, emotion, specific human interest (i.e. individuals), conflict and relevance.

This story was a cracker. The bald position was that:

- autism, a condition at least as frightening as, say, leukaemia, seems to be getting more common and we don't know why. Few readers, parents, journalists or editors understand what the condition is – ample mystery, therefore – but can imagine the devastation it causes

- it is often picked up and identified in toddlers at an age when they have recently had MMR, although a link has now been discredited

- there is an overwhelming human need for explanations even in the face of unalterable misery

- one small group of researchers on the basis of a tiny and, by common scientific consent, flawed study speculated on a link between autism and

MMR, and the journal publishing it put out a press release drawing attention to this[1]

- the entire weight of the rest of the world's researchers into the field said there was no link with existing evidence although they could always do more

- many parents, very few of whom had experience of the diseases that MMR prevents, then felt that there was a possible link between the vaccine and autism, and opted one way or another to 'play safe' and refuse the vaccine or give the components of it in separate doses.

My personal view is that there is a sense of a cover-up that has been further enhanced by previous incorrect advice presented as scientific failures, like the bovine spongiform encephalopathy (BSE) fiasco, and the failure of the former prime minister to give a ringing endorsement of the vaccine.

It was then easy to write or present stories with two sides. On the one hand dignified and serious scientists could say that no link was established (a yawning gap exists between 'not established' and 'not there') and that the speculative paper was 'almost certainly disproved' by many colossal studies from across the world. On the other hand a parade of parents whose children had autism proclaimed their belief that this might well have been caused by MMR – and if not that then what was it? The context of a culture to whom infectious diseases were not a perceived major threat, and vaccines feel artificial and scary, added weight to the distressed parents' side. The story then had all the needed elements of attraction: conflict (with and between scientists), emotion (involving children), relevance (your children) and mystery (what are these scientists on about?). Infuriated doctor-scientists hated their views being given equivalence to those of the unhappy families since they had opinions based on some impressive numbers. Journalists however felt they were giving balance, in much the same way as a victim of crime exhorting tougher sentencing is set against the judicial and criminology experts pointing out that tougher sentencing is ineffective. Eventually the clinicians twigged that they could not win this and stopped trying to persuade the public through the 'balanced' media and used other far more arduous methods, i.e. one-to-one discussions between the health visitors, GPs, community paediatric staff and their nervous patients. This has had a steady if limited success.

But why did the senior public health figures duck saying, in as many words, that the vaccine is safe? Not 'safe as far as we know' or 'safe except in unusual circumstances' or 'safe but...' anything – just 'safe'? There are few enough certainties in medicine but the evidence in favour of the universal use of this vaccine is one of them; the adverse event rate from it is known to be so rare that it is beyond the experience of whole colonies of primary care clinicians, which makes it much nearer the 'Will the sun rise tomorrow morning?' question than the 'Is this anaesthetic safe?' one.

The word scientist does not engender confidence in people. There are no clearly defined professional standards for someone who describes him or herself as a scientist. To be a doctor, and use the title, generally means that at some point in the holder's life some sort of quite high achievement was attained and some sort of standard accepted.* 'Scientist' gives a different image, not reliably including trust-worthy and benevolent features. A scientist is more likely to come over as scarily clever, naïve, single-minded and passionate about his or her field to the exclusion of others. And the mad scientist is an old cliché of Hollywood and cheap novels.

Furthermore, to a public yearning for certainty and with little training in how to assess degrees of it, scientists have often been 'wrong'. Examples of scientists being wrong are legendary; it was 'wrong' to declare that beef was completely safe some years ago† for instance. But the politicians and scientists in the beef scare were dealing with a situation (the emergence of a new disease, first in cattle and later as new-variant Creutzfeldt–Jakob disease (CJD) in humans) about which there really was uncertainty. Our knowledge base about these prion diseases was pitiful at the time and so it was disingenuous to try to say it was safe with a degree of certainty. They would have been better advised to say it was safe to eat beef so far as was understood at the time, and work was being done to eliminate even the theoretical risks. And, actually, that is what they did say but our memory is of patronising and didactic pronouncements.

The public, not wanting to make a difficult decision or hear news that they can't handle, finds it easy to discredit the argument using the run-over-by-a-bus principle. This works with the striking *non sequitur* of saying that they might as well carry on smoking, because they might be run over by a bus tomorrow. Arguments that at least 100,000 people die of smoking a year, and the numbers run over by buses are countable on the fingers of one hand, do not work in this situation.[2] The patient has taken an anti-science view and when the GP tries to correct this error by meeting it head on, we are met with denial rather than reason.

Similarly it is easy for the *non sequitur* to take root that because the advice given around beef was presented as a certainty but in fact was anything but, and it had been endorsed by hallowed scientists. Then of course any future scientific wisdom must be questionable at best.

GPs, holding a different image of what a scientist does and is, are rightly proud of their own scientific approach and by and large the senior bigwigs wheeled out by the Department of Health were termed 'leading scientist' or similar. Unfortunately with MMR they took the true scientists' view of 'almost certainty' as being intellectually accurate. What was needed with MMR, however, was the confidence to say that doctors do many things on the basis of probability, but the numbers in the MMR controversy are such that it counts as one of the treatments given that can be said to be of certain and absolute benefit.

In early 2006 the UK saw its first measles death for 14 years. The damage done by the controversy continues and we have had to be increasingly ingenious in countering it.[3]

---

* I know you can buy pseudo-qualifications but the point is about verifiable standards rather than quackery.

† Ironically, the judgement that beef is safe might well in fact have been the case, as the latest evidence is that the vCJD outbreak for which the beef was held responsible might be waning.

Dry doc

A physician at my medical school, whose undoubted skills in his field were quite overshadowed by the driest and most inappropriate bedside manner, was asked by a woman if she was going to die.

'All my patients die' he replied, in a husky tone that might have been well placed in a horror movie. But, after a brief dramatic pause, he then went on to explain that she need not fear that she would die just yet, or at least of the condition for which she had sought his help.

Literal certainty, then, can be the spectacularly wrong thing to give. The art of reassurance and appropriateness, discussed in later chapters, obviously involves knowledge of this rather human point.

There has been an assumption so far in this chapter, of course, that patients seek certainty from their clinical advisers. Is this so? It might be that patients are more sophisticated than we give them credit for, as in their own lives (unless perchance they are mathematicians) they are likely to be involved in some level of uncertainty and they know clinicians are only human. Perhaps it is a patronising generalisation to assume they want a straight and simple answer.

This has been looked at by Scott, a health economist from Aberdeen.[4] Instinct might suggest that the less well-educated and less well-read lower social classes might tolerate arguments about risks and estimates, which are laid out in many a clinical encounter, less well than those holding a more privileged rank in society. But a brief reflection suggests that requests for absolute truths in medicine come from the anxious and fraught types, who comprise a significant proportion of all strata; anxiety is somewhat independent of knowledge and the ability to process it. It has been suggested in fact that higher social classes are more likely to have medical tests for a given clinical situation (and so seek to reduce uncertainty) than those in lower classes. The lower social classes are more likely to get a prescription. However, many factors are going to be involved here, not least patient choice, financial influences (for patients outside the UK) and doctor characteristics – is it the type of GP who treats patients in higher socio-economic groups who tends to investigate more, or cope with uncertainty less?

We have to conclude that patients vary in their tolerance of medical uncertainty just as we know that doctors do. The lengths to which an individual will go to reduce uncertainty is not easily predicted from a knowledge of the background of the patient and attempts to do so can become paternalistic. The unconfident GP, fearing that patients might ask the impossible, tries not to allow them to present the question. The confident one knows when it is reasonable to be certain in the tone of his or her advice (MMR is safe) but will be comfortable reflecting back to patients when the issue is less clear (is it safe to have this hip replacement?) using the numbers and evidence he or she does possess. Sadly, many GPs and other clinicians will follow what is outwardly the confident approach but feel unconfident in it. These unhappy advisers are all too aware that sometimes the decision made by the patient will turn out to be wrong; some patients make an irrational choice, i.e. decline an operation or test when the benefits to most observers would seem to far outweigh the risks. Worse still of course some patients accept the small risk and fail to get away with it, so it is only human of the GP to wonder if he or she influenced them wrongly. Our confident colleague feels trained to discuss risks and let patients make choices, and he or she feels some weight of responsibility lifted from his or her shoulders as a result.[5]

As a further primary care example, there is a kind of fever phobia amongst the parents of children whose babies and toddlers catch an upper respiratory tract infection (URTI). The health beliefs behind this, of the dangers of fits, the need for early recognition of serious disease like meningitis, and the risk of cot death following an attack of the snuffles, have an underlying factual basis. Every casualty, NHS Direct and out-of-hours GP service is expected to cope with parents whose otherwise well children present with fevers often only for two, three or six hours, because of these worries. Here everyone seeks certainty, and the art of reassuring parents is an advanced skill (see Chapter 8). But when did parental coping skills drift away so much? When did the universal, homely scene of a child looking remotely peaky – especially if he or she has vomited a couple of times over Mum (or worse still, Dad) – become a medical emergency? Wrong questions, of course – the issue is why has responsibility shifted, and how can the GP handle it. Consider the presentation of such a feverish child, perhaps who has been sick once, or is a bit off colour but who was fine when he or she awoke this morning. The child has a bit of catarrh but no other clinical signs – our confident GP is more accurately here a clueless clinician, in that at this point at least they have to admit he or she is a long way from a diagnosis. The dilemma will be how much to share with the family, and how to do it. To use the word meningitis fearlessly and confidently but of course without certainty. It is not easy.

It seems obvious, to GPs as well as patients, that an early diagnosis of a treatable disease must be a good thing. There is indeed sound evidence that detecting CIN I on a smear carries a better prognosis than CIN III, and certainly invasive carcinoma. To be found to have a Dukes A bowel cancer, which has not by definition gone beyond the mucosa, brings the chance of cure towards 90 per cent whereas of course very few survive once the disease has metastasised (Dukes D). And the problem is that these conditions are not spotted in these early phases because of symptoms; we have to keep looking for them (or coming across them) with examinations of varying indignity and invasiveness or we won't know they are there. Unfortunately this appealing logic does not easily extend to all diseases.

There is continuing controversy over the value of mammography screening even though it certainly results in a number of presentations of breast cancer earlier than would have been discovered otherwise.[6] Yet many of these earlier presenting cases do not have an improved outcome compared with those who waited until the disease appeared clinically – i.e. some of these women survive longer with cancer because the disease was found earlier, but their death is not deferred. It is also true that another, smaller, proportion might have a better outcome (and the most recent studies are encouraging in this regard), so justifying the programme scientifically – perhaps two or three lives saved per thousand women irradiated, but at the cost of substantial morbidity in the large 'false positive' group. Politically of course the programme is untouchable whatever the evidence.

Another cancer that is worth understanding is prostate cancer. This is treatable, sometimes controllable, but is not essentially a curable disease. Because it affects men often of a considerable age many will die of other, unrelated, causes before the cancer caused any ill health, and so knowing that they have prostate cancer does not help in their medical care. The prostate-specific antigen (PSA) test is unfortunately neither sufficiently specific nor sensitive to make screening worthwhile, but many men nevertheless ask for it and it is incorporated in some private medical schemes' routine check-ups. No convincing evidence exists to suggest that the knowledge and treatment of this disease pre-symptomatically is worthwhile – which is not to say it won't eventually be forthcoming. The point is that a headlong dash for a certain answer to questions like 'Do I have a pre-symptomatic breast/prostate cancer?' does not necessarily lead to a better outcome.

Sudden death from a myocardial infarction (MI) is the first presentation of a significant proportion of cases of ischaemic heart disease. But exercise testing of asymptomatic patients in an attempt to spot the earliest signs of coronary artery disease also lacks specificity – it gives false positives. The airline industry has tried this screening for its pilots, whom it would prefer to survive until the plane lands. But it ended up grounding too many pilots with healthy hearts. The risk has to be assessed and acted on by population measures rather than individual ones – which is presumably why pilots look younger than they used to and now have names like Lee and Shane.

Discussing medical risk

> I never worry about seeing the doctor. To me it is just a matter of life
> and death but to him I know his whole career's at stake.

To have a risk there must be an unwanted outcome, or at least the failure of a wanted outcome. So the first problem might well be in defining this.

A middle-aged* patient who smokes describes a belly pain that seems to be, on careful listening and a bit of judicious but unrevealing prodding, possible dyspepsia of some sort: so the problem becomes what to do next. The GP reaches for NICE guidance, which says that the cut-off in the absence of alarm signs is age 55. Of course an older patient would have a significant risk of early stomach cancer that is well worth discovering, and therefore we know that endoscoping the older person is well worthwhile. A younger patient will have much less risk, though there were 100 cases of stomach cancer in patients under 40 last year in the UK. Our patient doesn't seem to fit into the rules; the GP still has a decision to make. Into the equations, but short of life/death issues, come issues of comfort and convenience. Endoscopies carry hassles like delays, time off work, and putting up with the symptoms until the result. They are not pleasant and there is a small but known complication rate. Furthermore, the community has to pay for this and we all have ethical responsibilities to the budget (whatever we think).

* Born before 1956

There is also the opportunity cost in that doing an unnecessary endoscopy denies someone else one, or delays it, and uses up a highly trained team of professionals' time that might be better spent on sicker people. And finally our patient will probably feel better immediately with a therapeutic dose of a proton pump inhibitor (PPI) of some sort. We could probably make him feel better tomorrow, and we all need grateful patients, even confident, happy GPs.

This decision is medically complex but could be broken down into useable components. There might be an optimum answer to this situation that weighs up the factors and comes up with the minimum risk and maximum benefit. One might hope that some kind of computer spreadsheet program might factor it all in and come up with an answer: better to scope or not? But the process of reaching that point is, perhaps thankfully, well beyond the possibility of any microchip to handle, because it is personally complex too.

The actual decision might be based on a lot of factors that the spreadsheet cannot factor in:

- what the clinician knows of the evidence around the issue and how sure he or she is of the boundaries of his or her own knowledge and expertise

- what the patient knows about it and how keen and able he or she is to learn

- the patient's tolerance of his or her symptoms

- the patient's tolerance of anxiety

- the patient's willingness to share his or her thoughts with advisers

- what personal experiences the GP (i.e. from handling other patients) and the patient bring to the discussion, probably also without actually saying so

- local resources

- what the other alternatives might be.

We are duty bound to gather as much evidence and information as easily practicable to inform us here – so the advising GP needs both self-awareness and a critical knowledge of the current literature. And there might be other ways of helping this patient, which might be deferring the decision but in fact is sensible, such as simple blood tests or therapeutic trials. The resource factor can be all-encompassing too, in that access to ultrasound for instance always generates a demand for ultrasound, because you might as well double check for gallstones.

What is difficult to gauge, as discussed above, is the patient's agenda before coming in to the room. Regrettably patients are unlikely to blurt it out, at least clearly and unambiguously because of the social inequality of the clinician–patient encounter, their fear of looking foolish or ignorant, the agenda not being in the form of conscious and articulate words or – heaven forbid – the GP not generating an open and safe environment in which they can speak and be heard. So it might well be best to discuss the options for our man and ask his opinion, using the information so far obtained to devise various options:

- we have a reasonable idea this is a benign form of dyspepsia and the first option is to wallop it with powerful drugs

- at the other extreme we could do an endoscopy with the following pros and cons locally, to more or less eliminate the remote risk of malignancy

- we could do other tests, which are easier but less definitive

- we could do one then the other

- we could get a second opinion because although I know about these things someone else might know more.

What might be needed is a way of discussing the virtues and drawbacks of each option in a manner that is both honest and understandable. There is quantitative information, any amount of it on many issues, but of course this never involves large numbers of patients in the exact medical and personal circumstances of our dyspeptic man. Qualitative information is powerful, especially when anecdotes heard by the patient are clearly given unreasonable weight – 'my mate had an endoscopy and said he felt sick for weeks after'. The clinician will find the patient's mate's view carries great store even after the most careful deconstruction, nevertheless, but it must be helpful to the clinician to at least understand this influence. Some patients are very visual and understand drawings and graphs more than words, and so many of our desks are scattered with scraps of drawings of human bits, or simplistic graphs (all too often with a drug advertisement along the x axis).

What he might want to know is our opinion on the best option of those given, and the GPs have to decide whether they have a good enough opinion to be worth influencing the patient powerfully. This is where the knowing what one knows is crucial. The nervous patient might well feel that, if the doctor says he or she is not sure, then there might be a cleverer clinician around somewhere who is certain. This of course is possible and a way out of the impasse for both parties. But it is unsatisfactory for many situations because the application of the current best evidence to an individual situation is a matter of judgement more than knowledge here. Delegating to other doctors whenever there is doubt is not the sign of a confident GP and not what we should be doing automatically.

The question is who should be that judge, and the GP's art is to get the patient to take that role. And doctors have to do this feeling comfortable, and secure in themselves, rather than fearing that they cannot trust the patient's judgement. That way the patient might weigh in his or her unspoken issues – perhaps unwanted outcomes that are not the kinds of measurable physical harm that the GP has carefully described, but more psycho-social issues. Perhaps the disapproval of their relatives if they were to decline investigation, or particular problems with work or perhaps the need for denial within the patient – none of these is necessarily spoken aloud.

Patients can become qualified to decide about this endoscopy in their own case, and the confident GP should agree with them, whichever way they jump. This contrasts with the MMR decision, where the doctor can give a clear, unambiguous answer based on knowledge and experience. This decision sharing works where the GP is genuinely happy with there being more than one option – what was called by Elwyn 'equipoise'[5] – and has the skills to be visibly neutral.

The salesman again

The pharmaceutical representative is a fascinating specimen to study in a book on confidence and certainty in clinical practice. They are trained to appear, or be, confident (possibly the same thing) and exude health, good looks, charm and of course generosity, albeit within industry guidelines. The amount spent on marketing drugs to UK doctors is over £10,000 a year per doctor. Some of this goes on sponsorship of meetings of educational value, or conferences, or 'conferences'.... Some is spent on the publication and distribution of magazines and such – up to several kilos a week per GP – and some on the representatives (reps). The reps are not badly paid and have perks, even whilst working hard, with some pretty unsocial hours. There is some competition for these jobs and the successful rep has to be reasonably educated. And though not strictly on a commission-based income, they are like missionaries for their product.

The fervour with which they can deliver a sales patter must come from the heart. It is not subtle, particularly, but is quietly passionate. They succeed because they bring confidence to the decision-making GP who is feeling battered by information and demands that appear to conflict and be irreconcilable.

This is not to say it is not a good sales pitch to introduce uncertainty.

- We are all convinced of the value in many circumstances of statins, but the one you are using is not backed up by as good an authority or study as our one.

- We all worry about litigation but our drug has a proven safety record (unstated but implying not so sure about your current one).

- We all worry about cost and I am pleased to say this drug is now the most cost-effective in its class (not the cheapest – calculation involves various assumptions such as saved admissions to hospital through greater efficacy).

These claims are backed with graphs whose origin is rarely at zero, but which are very pretty. They are backed with references that the doctor might not recognise and approving asides about a respected colleague's prescribing of said product. And the name is mentioned lots of times.

The anxious doctor is thereby offered a way out of his or her distress, namely prescribing the drug in question, and by this means it is understood that the sun will rise in the morning again.

So we have looked at how the definition of certainty needs to be a bit more flexible provided the mathematicians around will forgive us. We need to accept that in a number of circumstances the GP must not be afraid to be certain where he or she has reason to be so, because expressing academic uncertainty purely for philosophical completeness results in poor individual decisions.

We also need a sense of judgement about how much use the elimination of uncertainty might be, even for life-threatening conditions. This requires a good knowledge of current evidence, and an ability to critique it.

But as GPs we have to understand what science is and where it can help, then we need to use it – though the definition of a scientist needs tightening up. We are the most scientific of all the average citizen's regular advisers and should trumpet this triumph where we can. Yet because the tidy application of scientifically demonstrated wisdom to an individual case is the unusual rather than common scenario, we must delegate to – or at least share with – patients much of the decision making. Patients might well use yardsticks that we are not happy with, or evidence that we do not trust, to make those decisions, but still we must see ourselves as facilitators not parents, or we'll worry too much.

And this requires using a set of skills that to those new to primary care feels threatening in both training and application.

Conclusion

We need to accept that certainty is a rare thing in life, never mind medicine, but some risks are proven to be so remote that they ought to be totally discounted, and we should be strong in doing so. We need to share all other risks with the patient and let them carry this burden with us. They can do it with some careful discussion with their GP. A change of mind in the light of new evidence is not intellectual weakness, but some advice won't ever change and we should challenge the anti-science approach robustly.

References

1. Wakefield A, Murch SH, Anthony A, *et al*. Ileal-lymphoid-nodular hyperplasia, non-specific colitis, and pervasive developmental disorder in children *Lancet* 1998; **351**: 637–41 [retraction in Murch SH, Anthony A, Casson DH, *et al. Lancet* 2004; **6**; 363(9411): 750; PMID: 15016483].

2. Bogardus ST, Holmboe E, Jekel JF. The perils, pitfalls and possibilities in talking about medical risk *Journal of the American Medical Association* 1999; **281**: 1037–41.

3. Wallace C, Leask J, Trevena LJ. Effects of a web based decision aid on parental attitudes to MMR: a before and after study *British Medical Journal* 2006; **332**: 146–8.

4. Scott A, Shiell A, King M. Is GP decision making associated with the patient's socio-economic status? *Social Science and Medicine* 1996; **42**: 35–46.

5. Elwyn G, Edwards A, Kinnersley P, *et al*. Shared decision making and the concept of equipoise: the competences of involving patients in healthcare choices *British Journal of General Practice* 2000; **50**: 892–7.

6. Gøtzsche PC, Olsen O. Is screening for breast cancer with mammography justifiable? *Lancet* 2000; **355**: 129–34.

CHAPTER 6

The use and misuse of personal clinical experience

Good judgement usually comes from experience. Experience often comes from bad judgement.
(Alan Gress)

This chapter discusses several issues. The first is the way in which anecdotal and individual clinical experience alters our behaviour and perception of risk. The second issue is observing the manner in which GPs might use clinical experience to identify their own educational needs, again endeavouring to balance appropriately.

Referral behaviour, learning and experience are looked at.

We also discuss getting patients to tell us more than their personal clinical story and even, in context, the diagnosis.

The problem in medicine is that the consequences of the badly thought out decision might be grim, and not just for the doctor. Conscientious clinicians find themselves burdened with a degree of guilt and a tendency to mentally revisit the problem to check that everything they could reasonably do has been done. They have a physical timescale to do this, and physical constraints, but mentally they can chew on matters well into the night and weekend, and indeed well past the deadline for action, making them ruminate aimlessly. This is human but very counter-productive.

This discussion however is about the clash between common sense, learning, anecdote and experience, and how any given piece of clinical wisdom is modified, or even battered, by personal factors. The effect of encountering problems and accumulating a memory bank of frightening anecdotes is to impede sound decision making, so the more experienced doctor, paradoxically, might struggle to make balanced decisions.[1]

The old on-call rota system for junior doctors was simple enough, we all thought. On a one-in-three, daytimes roughly ran from 8 a.m. to 5 or 6 p.m., plus every third night and weekend on call. Therefore the doctor might be on duty from Saturday morning at 8 a.m. to Monday afternoon at 6 or so. Different jobs carried different burdens of calls so the obstetric unit was notorious for only allowing minimal sleep, as was the medical unit, but the dermatology job was as quiet as a cemetery. But try as those who were junior doctors in the 1970s and 1980s did, neither parents, nor some non-medical friends nor sometimes even nurses, actually believed this was what happened, that this was how we worked. It was beyond sense and experience that anyone would be expected to function, let alone save lives for 32 or even 54 hours in a row. This was because, although the parents, friends and colleagues from other professions were reasonable folk and faced with a manifestly unreasonable piece of information, it is sometimes best dealt with by assuming you have misunderstood it. Surely the doctors were exaggerating? No, this was the clash between common sense and actual experience, and the only useful learning to come from it was that doctors discovered they are not always believed.

The virtue of this heroic induction into life as a junior doctor, in so far as there was any, was that the experience gained was intense and broad, rapidly developing the doctor into a more worldly and skilled clinician who has a good chance of having seen it all before.

A lesser virtue perhaps was the one of continuity of care, fondly thought to be the necessary precondition for a doctor to gain longitudinal experience of the course of patients' illnesses. (However, modern shift systems do not make for many more handovers of care than the old one-in-threes and, in any case, patients in hospital now turn over so swiftly that the patients with, say, pneumonia or a hernia or a fractured hip only spend a minority of the time that they are ill actually on the acute hospital site.) Continuity is now even more the preserve of primary and community care, and a proportion of outpatient work. Only GPs and some consultants who are well settled in their posts actually have the pleasure of seeing the patient for more than a brief interval, and knowing the patient when he or she is not especially poorly. Indeed, knowing them as ordinary people.

So did the clamour of being 'on take' for acute cases, dramatically ill people and opportunities for macho interventions help us become better clinicians in due course, simply by sheer volume of patient experience? Or did the culture of the fabulous anecdote and extreme experience distort our view of which options might be available for our patients? We don't know.

The value of inexperience

Teenagers' sense of certainty is magnificent. They have the ability to cut the fluff away from the complex reasoning of their elders and form an opinion based on far less information than adults are comfortable with, which might be viewed as a desirable quality. It is a skill that we lose as we get older and that adds value to teenagers' lives. For instance, in choosing what to eat or wear or see at the cinema it seems the average teenager uses a set of parameters – freely admitted to be driven by the moment's fashions – and measures the proposal against those. So their clothes might be less than ideal for the weather, but that is not the parameter by which they are judged. Their food is perhaps unbalanced and restrictive, consisting of pizzas and, well, pizzas, but it is the one that gives the immediate gratification – the parameter food is judged by, not the serum vitamin level. And the film or concert to be attended might be an appalling, overrated, over-priced noisy pain, but it is a fashionable one and that differentiates them from the older generation – and these kinds of parameters have priority. Even bigger issues, like choice of career or further education, and whether to work for exams, are likely to be decided on what to an older adult seem simpler or even naïve criteria – like where the boyfriend is headed, the attractiveness of a website, or if the hassles of early-morning lectures can be avoided by one course of action or another.

69

And teenagers then remain cool and relaxed, it seems. How do they do this? Is it that they make decisions on thin ground and then don't review them, happily more prepared to face the consequence of a decision that turned out wrong, than to indulge in persistent angst? Or do they simply not know better because of a sheer lack of life experience and so lack the imagination to see what could go wrong? Perhaps the teenager has the sense of a safety net from the consequences of life's poorer decisions, a cushion ensuring nothing can go totally wrong in the end. But, nonetheless, can older adults learn from them?

Younger doctors, viewed by their grey-haired colleagues without much evidence as being less dedicated and committed than their elders were, might be seen to have some of the skills of decision making seen in the teenager. There is the paucity of experience. For instance, being involved in the management of a couple of ectopic pregnancies might allow their confidence to build in the care of women with unexplained vaginal bleeding and pain – and so the young doctor or nurse feels able to 'spot' the worrisome case from the stack of patients presenting with such symptoms. And they feel faintly confused that their community colleagues are unable to do the same assessment and keep sending such patients into hospital, and even more confused that their boss thinks that this is quite sensible. The boss, of course, can remember some difficult cases and near misses that the young clinician has only read about and so they are less real. Yet, objectively, the young doctor (or nurse) is going to be right a lot more than most of the time. They will have for the time being pretty sharp clinical skills in this one field, and if they know the literature and learn to create effective safety nets then they can safely send home a proportion of patients whom the nervous boss might have kept in for observation for a day or two. A few might have to return, but the application of protocol-driven care with good clinical skills will ensure this is a minority. The boss probably rarely sees such cases and is no longer perhaps the expert.

Good luck and judgement

In striving for more accuracy the tendency can be to move away from the use of clinical skills and towards investigation. When a GP has his or her clinical skills apparently confounded by an unexpected but important X-ray or lab result they have a sense of this being a near miss. Lucky we did that X-ray, eh? The problem is that the next patient is also assumed to have a silent killer disease until proved otherwise. The reflection that in the patient last week who, for instance, did turn out to have had a silent myocardial infarction (MI) we did actually have enough suspicion to do the electrocardiogram (ECG) or admit him or her – the patient was a bit more breathless perhaps, or pale or slightly feverish even in the absence of chest signs – is mentally discounted. It is as if the patient has been managed by a GP split into two individuals. One is cautious, organised the X-ray, got the diagnosis (and is thus better), and the other is the low-tech partner, prone to gut feelings and hasty decisions, and a clinician we do not want to be. But the truth is that the absence of clinical signs is a significant finding too, the weight attached to the presence or absence of them is a clinical skill in itself and the patient was not in any danger all along – merely that on this occasion the clincher came from the test not the examination. We fear being the GP who misses things, especially physical diagnoses, as Balint pointed out 50 years ago.[2] The fear is sometimes misplaced, though, for we have a tendency to listen to our technocratic side without giving credit to that part of ourselves which actually listened to the patient.

So what is normal checking behaviour? Is there a judgement to be made about the number of sources of information we require before we accept something as an established fact? Trainee journalists are advised to get two independent sources for the pertinent 'facts' written in their copy. Psychiatrists might feel that going back to check that the door was locked properly is acceptable two or three times but four or more is pathological checking behaviour. The literature in unclear.

The dangers of using clinical experience to inform educational needs

Much of the continuing education of doctors could be seen as providing a poor experience in confidence building. There are many ways in which education of doctors unwittingly increases the sense of unease, occurring at all stages of the educational cycle.

The major advance in the last decade of change in the medical educational world has been the idea that learning needs to be personalised and focused on the aims of the learner. So the concept of the top-down dictation of the agenda for learning by authorities like college tutors and institutions and consultants, often delivered in undemanding lectures to large groups, has been abandoned. This is clearly an improvement but in some ways at a cost to self-confidence and contentment.

In looking at their educational needs GPs are encouraged to try to assess, as clearly and objectively as they can, where they have gaps. This might be by the route of jotting down the patient's unmet needs and doctor's educational needs (PUNS and DENS), which means one identifies consciously where one feels to have failed a patient.[3] It might be more formal assessments like exams and tests, looking like the school teacher using mock public exams to root out the detail where the pupil failed the questions. Clearly patients complain, colleagues give feedback and audits might point to deficiencies in performance, all of which gets placed in the portfolio, if the GP is conscientious or hounded about it. Of course the upbeat feedback should be placed in there too, with notes from happy patients and positive results from tests of how good one is, but real life will tend to lead to these being undermined, or overwhelmed, by the lists of negativity.

Greater awareness of one's faults by this means is bound to increase anxiety.[4] Whilst pricking the bubble of inappropriate self-confidence, in other words arrogance, is necessary, the tools we have to do it with are crude. They will sometimes harm a GP's appropriate self-confidence. A PUN might lead one to conclude that the ability to manage that type of case is poor, whereas the case in question was odd and atypical; audits are very open to different interpretations and explanations; exams test the ability to do exams.

The classic dilemma for the examiner in setting fact-testing exams like multiple-choice questions (MCQs) lies in the temptation to restrict questions to those based on absolutely verifiable data. '50 per cent of men over 85 have histological evidence of Ca prostate. True/False.' The correct figure might be 30 per cent, but this is a useless 'fact'. The important clinical issue is that a large proportion of elderly men have histological evidence of Ca prostate. Exactly how large is unimportant to most of the usual examinees and all of the patients. But by creating the expectation in doctors that they have to know this stuff, and proving to them they don't, all we do is make them feel incompetent, which might be very far from the truth. It is fair to say there is now a flood of literature about more carefully assessing educational need,[5] and greater efforts are made by the examining authorities to improve the process of identifying the truly competent (e.g. nMRCGP).

But the unconfident GP will still have little faith in the process and might well be tempted to commit the minimum effort to the needs assessment segment of the education cycle.

Using the tough case constructively

How can we learn to use clinical experience positively without examples of problems crushing us by leaping into our consciousness all the time? The patient whose dizzy turns were found to be early Addison's disease and the patient whose painful knee was found to be an osteosarcoma will never be forgotten but they cannot be allowed to control the way we look after patients with dizzy turns (with 20 causes more common than Addison's) and persisting aching knees (of whom we would have to irradiate 100,000 to find the next osteosarcoma).

The identification of the problem has to be the start. The GP has to identify that when he or she spots a patient's unmet need (or a critical event) a whole set of reasons might be behind that failure. These are listed on Table 6.1.

Table 6.1: Why were the patient's needs not met?

Type of case	*Educational response*
The doctor did not know the best way of managing the condition that the patient presented with, or the optimum strategy for resolving the medical complaint	Represents true educational need and the doctor has an obligation to seek these out and meet them. This might mean using considerable resources
The doctor usually knows what to do but the patient was atypical, which was a surprise. However, this might have been realised earlier	These types of case warrant some learning but briefly and opportunistically, because they are interesting and of conceivable importance in the future
As above, but the patient was highly atypical and this could not have been anticipated	Whilst interesting there is no educational need here
The failure to meet the patient's needs was due to another part of the system for which the GP was not responsible	This is where the concept of clinical governance arises, and represents management and political need as much as clinical
The system failed to meet the needs of the patient because at that point, of necessity, there were different priorities. No one failed to do anything but they were needed elsewhere	As above, only even more starkly
The patient confounded attempts at help because he or she had a different agenda, which might not include getting better. They might even need to be ill	Sometimes you can do nothing about it

The educational need of the doctor has to be teased out, because the single case is not necessarily helpful. The GP has an obligation to decide if the problem is the first of the categories on Table 6.1 but by checking on his or her abilities by some other means, and if found to have a significant gap, then of course allocating significant resource to plugging it. A review of similar cases, perhaps, or a chat with a colleague or using a CD-ROM program if a sensible one exists.

So if a doctor feels that an unfortunate case might point to a draughty gap in his or her knowledge base, he or she should use other assessment methods to confirm or refute the feeling. The new GP curriculum on the RCGP website is a good place for evaluating relevance of a topic area.

Using the dull case constructively

A less threatening approach to identifying one's needs might be to think about patients whom one has encountered and found the experience to be dull, boring or irritating. This is different from the obvious pick-out-the-mistakes method because here one assumes the patient was dealt with well and would give a different account of the interaction. But given that all clinicians face routine and repetitive cases, or frustrating and long-term problems that they at times do not look forward to seeing, then a perfectly reasonable educational need might be construed as 'learning to enjoy (whatever sort of case) again'. This need might be met by looking at the recent literature, meeting an enthusiast, sharing the hassle of such cases with like-minded colleagues. Or looking at where within the case there is a lack of sparkle – possibly the communication methods used, or the unimaginative therapy options of which one knows. It might lead to an examination of the healthcare system that seems to send so many such cases to them, or appears to, or the learning need might evolve into exploring better ways of delegating. All of this might spring from looking at the GP's daily grind rather than the crises.

Confident choices of educational activity

Where there is an apparent gap in knowledge GPs must decide if filling the gap is going to be:

- important, useful for their work or their goals like exams

- relevant, likely to be needed for patient care or other responsibilities

- proportionate, i.e. will the time taken to gain this knowledge or skill be in a sensible ratio to the frequency of using it?

- is there another way round, for instance instead of learning what to do in situation A, perhaps the learning should be in knowing who locally can deal with situation A so one can smoothly refer or delegate?

After all this rationalisation, busy GPs will still have to admit that they feel uncertain in certain aspects of the job, which they will need to be more confident in. Here they will need to check, preferably with someone else, if the problem is ability or lack of confidence. The planning phase of the cycle will go wrong if the lack of confidence is not spotted. It will also go wrong if the problem is labelled as 'just lacking confidence' and dismissed, since the GP's approach to the patient might remain less than ideal just from that.

Constraints on meeting the educational need – and the luck of unplanned learning

After working on his or her educational needs and gaps the GP has to plan what to do to fill them. This might be simple on the surface but the barriers to provision are considerable, and even with a dialogue with the best of mentors there will be problems. Different learners will prefer different methods and the unconfident might well opt for undemanding, spongy methods like listening to the words of experts and sitting in with the wise and worldly. The educational establishments now feel this is demonstrably ineffective. The billed wizard might not be such an expert, and might have his or her own beliefs and unspoken or spoken agendas. Most importantly, if the learner is not actively joining in, he or she is unlikely to be taking much on board. So a GP sitting in with a gynaecology clinic might enjoy the dialogue and discussion of some cases but the case mix is not likely to be very relevant to him or her, the setting alien and the style inappropriate. Or a doctor going to a conference lecture on the pathology of a rare condition or the latest trial evidence of a new drug might appreciate the stimulation – so making it a worthwhile venture in itself – but is unlikely to find the content correlating well with the identified gaps on his or her learning plan. Finally, we all work with constraints like time schedules so when a really useful learning opportunity arises it might be impossible to attend because a colleague is on holiday or it's your day to do the school run. The solution of dedicating working time to the pursuit of education is admirable, but all GPs find it to be squeezed too easily. Having arrived at the educational event, fired up and excited, the doctor might yet be faced with disappointment. The drive behind providing educational events is often commercial in its broadest sense. The pharmaceutical industry might well have heavily sponsored its pro-drug speaker even if he or she sticks to within industry guidelines; a discussion on care of post-myocardial infarction patients might spend ages on the management of hypercholesterolaemia and little on exercise programmes. Many an individual, or trust or other NHS body, seeking to promote use of a new service or facility will get themselves on the lecture and seminar sheet. Small-group discussions that are well facilitated might be less prone to the organiser's biases but facilitation is a rare skill. The real benefit of the event is shown by the conversation back at the workface next day, when the refreshed attendee is asked how it went. The food was good, we reflect, and we met X, Y and Z and caught up with them – their team/practice/service does this…. And that…. The educational content might be mentioned too, if there is time.

The cycle will be completed by an evaluation of whether the gaps identified previously have now been filled. This too is a dispiriting activity, so demoralising that little emphasis is placed on it by most GPs despite the obvious need for an evidence base for our own learning and the requirement of General Medical Council (GMC) revalidation etc. The tendency to adopt a different method of evaluation, something dangerously close to gut feeling, is strong.

The educational cycle should move up a gear now to fill the gap, and it is not my intention to discuss in any further detail how this is best done; a bucketful of literature awaits the reader.[5] Suffice to remark that GPs should not be defeated by poorly directed educational events, and indeed attend them without guilt for the social interaction. But they know their real learning is likely to be in private or in a small circle, and hard work.

The unconfident GP might tend to tell him or herself that reading a lot, and attending 'Events', will be the way to tackle the nervousness he or she feels. When this fails, the tendency is to increase the dose of the medicine – read more and lose more time to 'Events', whereas the fact might be that he or she is tackling the issue as a knowledge problem rather than a confidence one.

Referrals and cross-referrals

There exists in medicine a rule saying we should never criticise a referral. This makes some sense as a criticism is likely to be based on ignorance – alleging that it was unnecessary, for instance, when the full facts of the situation are not known. The secondary sector knows that it will get a great deal more than inappropriate referrals dumped on them if they make a fuss.

Naturally it is as well to remember that referrals justify a service even when it has problems meeting present commitments so can be seen as a kind of currency in negotiations between managers and directorates. Turning them down is not in the unit's interest, even more so following the changes to how funds move from April 2006 (Payment by Results).

But the reasons for a referral are not simple[6] and need to be understood by all sides.[7] Superficially people like politicians categorise referrals as all being needed because they are the difficult cases. It seems one doctor or clinician passes a case onto another because:

- the patient needs a technical procedure for treatment, e.g. hernia repair, an enema, electroconvulsive therapy (ECT), angioplasty. The referrer is aware of what needs to be done

- the patient needs the expert opinion of someone who specialises in that problem and has particular experience. The referrer might not be aware of what would be ideal, and hopes the new doctor or clinician will take over management. The referrer might also know that the specialist to whom the patient is being sent has a particular personal or research interest in such cases

- the patient needs, or might need, hospital or technical investigation not available to the referrer for further evaluation of the case to reach a diagnosis, e.g. computed tomography (CT) scan, infertility tests, psychological tests

- the patient demands a second opinion and has stuck to that, implying a degree of lost faith in the GP or first clinician, not always unjustified

- the patient needs the expertise of a different doctor for advising the GP on clinical management, e.g. palliative care, dyspepsia, memory loss, arthritis. But the referrer GP expects to remain in charge

- the GP has become exhausted and needs to share the burden, e.g. many chronic illnesses – back pain, atypical or chronic abdominal or chest symptoms. The referrer needs a break but expects the patient back in due course.

The first four are examples not of sharing care but passing it all on; the patient is put in the hands of the more appropriate doctor for care until such time as the patient is relieved of his or her problem (see Appendix 1). This is the patient pathway beloved of on-the-ball managers and ambitious politicians, and can work very smoothly for a range of situations. That many a patient strays from the path by having slightly different circumstances than foreseen in the pathway document, and clutter the path with a range of coexisting physical or psychosocial issues, serves to make life more complex but also more interesting.

The penultimate reason for referral shows the desire of many in primary and community care, which is to consult the consultant (whether from a medical or nursing background) for advice and then decide whether to take it. Not all the parties, certainly including the patient, explicitly understand this, and much of the tension around referrals arises when advice is not acted upon or even seems to be ignored. Who is carrying the can after it goes wrong, when A asks B about C and then ignores the answer? Is it the adviser B who was too diffident and unclear in giving a suggestion about the best course of action, the patient C who might be behaving in a rather active and difficult way rather than the passive and co-operative manner that is so much easier? Or is it the referrer A who appears to have wasted everyone's time? This failure of communication around the point of the exercise makes the professional parties involved nervous, especially next time over patient D. So the GP can deal with this by several strategies, all involving better communication between all concerned. This might start with sharing all the information, including inter-professional correspondence, with the patient. Then the goals of the referral would be clear, e.g. 'Please advise how this skin disease should be managed and I will happily carry on from there' or 'Please could you suggest what non-surgical options there might be for this patient's back pain'. If the goal is 'Please take over the care of this patient's back' then it might be best to say so; then the physiotherapist or whoever is being approached knows where he or she is. Once seen it is very effective for the adviser to write a letter back saying 'I have seen Ms X and she has the following options for her rash that she is thinking about. If the chosen option is the one needing hospital facilities then please contact me again.' And nowadays all copied to the patient.

There is then no confidence-sapping sense of mystery around the correspondence and opinions, and the patient's control of the problem reduces the doctor's vulnerability and keeps expectations explicit.

The final reason noted for making a referral is no more than the need to be given respite from the problems of a chronically symptomatic patient who perhaps him or herself struggles to cope. An experienced GP might be able to say that he or she has got to this point and it is at present beyond him or her to do any more. Hanging on to the patient for ever – by arranging endless reviews at intervals of weeks or months – is justified internally by the kindly doctor on the grounds that it is supportive. As indeed it might be, although the same clinician has an ethical duty to remember the opportunity cost of time given to such patients. Here the actual reasons and expectations of referral are sometimes best written between the lines, although honesty can work. A well-run pain clinic, the entire psychotherapy department, the community occupational therapist's and the diabetic service and others, all run this kind of support mechanism. It is for colleagues who are weary of individual patients and need someone else to keep the problem ticking over, with some tinkering, for a spell before they go back to the GP and the primary healthcare team. These services will find things to do, and might occasionally surprise the referrer with an effective intervention. But they have to pass the patient back eventually because this respite care is only a small part of their job, obviously the larger being their more medically effective activities.

An unspoken reason for referrals, but which certainly occurs, is idleness. At its worst this might be a GP who knows that with some extra effort he or she could deal with a case but cannot be bothered to do so. Sometimes advice by telephone by a GP for a patient to go to A&E, or advice by an A&E clinician to go to a GP, might fall into this category. But the laziness might mask poor communication skills, too, in failing to find out what the patient wants and how the patient sees his or her role in helping attain this. We are all guilty of this at times. Ironically, by their nature such situations have a habit of rebounding on the clinician, who ends up dealing with it anyway, the tenaciousness of patients being quite wondrous.

So the conclusion about the experiences gained from the frustrations of referrals, and the way it is hard to gauge effective feedback and learning from them, is that there is a danger of the GP's confidence being assaulted. On the one hand all referrals will be justified by the person to whom they are sent, but on the other the referrer might have a sense that they have too low a threshold or, like the patient who is fearful of the accusation of malingering, might be thought to be lazy. The referrer seeks reassurance from the wrong person – the patient, who likes the attention, or the other clinician, who needs to be needed. GPs have to learn to evaluate their reasons for referring and be explicit, to compare only with GPs doing the same job, and to be sure of their desire to do the best for the patient.

Asking the patient for a diagnosis

If we have a patient with a pain in the chest, which hurts when he or she breathes, there is a possibility that the problem is a pulmonary embolus (PE) and we have to exclude it. The patient's age, predisposing factors, and past medical history will be needed to start to make the judgement. Then there are the particular details of the history in this case and the findings on examining the chest. In primary care or A&E work, in at least nine out of ten cases of pleuritic pain, we will conclude that the patient has a low risk of a PE at this point, but in only two or three of these nine will we have a clear diagnosis of, say, injury or pleurisy.

We might go and sit down whilst the patient gets dressed and give ourselves a few moments of thinking time, because we now have a difficult decision. We might very well go and wash our hands again, to give ourselves even more time, and just to be sure we have not become contaminated from examining the patient (but naturally not washing more than twice).

If there is no clear diagnosis then three options beckon: arrange for a fancy investigation because the risk feels high; arrange symptomatic treatment; or look more closely at the patient again. In the latter group we might think it worth checking for an obvious leg deep-vein thrombosis (DVT) (guiltily but not logically thinking we should have done this first time), knowing they are not usually obvious. We might do pulse oximetry, or an ECG or a chest X-ray if available as near-patient tests, but none of these is going to be conclusive. A therapeutic trial of a non-steroidal anti-inflammatory drug (NSAID) might help, perhaps with a nurse or telephone review in a few hours. And we might have another careful listen to the history and the chest, to see if any shafts of light shine from there. Some of these devices might help us with the decision, and reduce the uncertainty. Others won't and some patients will still leave us feeling unsure.

The final option we could consider is asking the patient what he or she thinks is the problem.[8] Even confident doctors find this difficult because it feels like an abrogation of responsibility.

'What do you think is happening here?' with the emphasis on the 'you' can come over as a bit stark and blunt. There is the risk that the patient will take the opportunity to remind the GP of his or her traditional role in answering that question, and of the doctor feeling mildly rebuked or even affronted.

'I was wondering what your thoughts on the cause of this pain were...' with a trailing end is more inviting and open, though many patients will not feel able to share their fears.

Another tactic might be to admit a degree of defeat, reasoning aloud, 'The pain is not typical of any particular chest problem and examining you I can find no unusual sounds in your chest.' Many a patient thinks of auscultation as the only useful part of the examination ceremony. 'Did you have any feelings about the cause of the pain?' This starts the idea of a partnership, and at least partial ownership of the pain by its victim.

And the situation will arise when the pain has elements of psycho-social or psychosomatic origins. Many doctors are nervous of proposing this as a source of a pain that might also have a possibly serious physical basis. But it needs to be done to prevent hopeless over-investigation and wild goose chases. So, in asking the patient his or her view on the cause of the pain it can help to say 'Do you think this is a physical or a psychological stress-type pain?' perhaps prefacing it with a single sentence explaining that sometimes such symptoms can have a 'nervous' basis. The antennas need to be on maximum sensitivity here because a patient will answer, possibly obliquely,

- 'Actually I think this might be stress related, because....' In this case the GP might not be home and dry but at least has a way forward and an umbrella

- 'I have no reason to be stressed, really....' Here the patient is ducking the issue but not keen on the idea of 'nerves' and will need reassuring that he or she is believed. The biggest fear, after all, is the accusation of being a wimp or malingerer

- 'No, I am sure it is physical....' When the patient is definite about this, even when the GP strongly suspects the symptom to have at least a major psychological element, the only way forward for now will be the pursuit of physical disease. But the seed is planted, and some time later it might germinate.

This shows that in asking the patient for an opinion on his or her health, the answer is important and must be seen to be acted on. Even if, later, the strategy changes.

So our patient with chest pain might have a pertinent view, an approach that helps us along. We might be drawn into a discussion about a family member's woes or some other diversion. Or, for instance, he or she might have a strong view on the need for a 'scan' or might add in a bit of history not thought to be pertinent until that point, like a sporting injury. Coaxing the patient into sharing opinions should empower the doctor, because it is sharing the uncertainty. The GP will then be able to go on to sharing options for what to actually do about it all, genuinely interested in the patient's view.

Building the bridge

The card game bridge – bear with me here – is played with two pairs of players conventionally denoted N, S, E and W. The pack is fully distributed and each player has to decide where the strengths and weaknesses of his or her 13 cards are. Then, working with his or her partner opposite, using an elaborate coding system, explore what might be a workable contract, i.e. how many tricks (played as in whist) they could make between them if a particular suit are trumps. Points are awarded if a contract is bid and then met, and of course to the opposition if the contract is not met. The bidding is very sophisticated and many deductions can be made from each piece of information, and of course the opposing pair gleans some oblique information about where the strong cards are from the information in a bid. The idea is to minimise uncertainty, so the team going for their contract is, once the playing starts, not taken by surprise, e.g. by not having sufficient trumps. But it is also about judging risk because the more lucrative contract is not made without a bit of a gamble. One of the biggest risks comes from the distribution of cards – for instance, one might know that the opposition has five of the 13 trump cards, and hope they are split 3:2 between the players, which makes winning tricks easier. And this is in fact more likely than 4:1 or 5:0 – but you don't play the game long before you unexpectedly get that worst distribution. And usually lose the contract as a result. Tradition has it that a brief reflective period follows the contract to justify the bid, or learn from the play. The blame for failure is important, because on the one hand one can fault the poor distribution rather than poor bidding and play, but on the other one can root out some learning points. The behaviour of the bidders next time is thus affected by the cards they hold, the points they need, what has happened in the recent past, the attitude to risk of all the other players and who got criticised last time.

Who feels lucky? It's only a game. But if the parallel is with the doctor and patient versus their diseases and problems, then it is vital for both to remember that sometimes you can do everything right, and it still goes wrong...and there is no learning to be gained here, because the original plan was optimum.

Conclusions

This chapter admires the abilities of teenagers to make decisions. It briefly explores why single adverse encounters seem to alter our behaviour disproportionately. After all, sometimes you do everything right and yet everything goes wrong. We start to consider involving the patient more in the dialogue and even ask his or her opinion. The actual words the clinician uses are delicate, but worth practising. We look a little at using experience to inform our educational needs. Finally, we explore the value of sharing patient care with colleagues and of having explicit goals when we do so.

References

1. Peile E, Carter Y. Selecting and supporting contented doctors *British Medical Journal* 2005; **330**: 269–70.

2. Balint M. *The Doctor, His Patient and the Illness* London: Pitman, 1957.

3. Eve R. *PUNs and DENs: discovering learning needs in general practice* [Radcliffe Professional Development Series] Abingdon: Radcliffe Publishing, 2003.

4. Davis DA, Mazmanian PE, Fordis M, *et al*. Accuracy of physician self-assessment compared with observed measures of competence: a systematic review *Journal of the American Medical Association* 2006; **296**: 1137–9.

5. Graham D, Chambers R, Wakeley G, *et al*. *Appraisal for the Apprehensive: a guide for doctors* Abingdon: Radcliffe Publishing, 2002.

6. Faulkner A, Mills N, Bainton D, *et al*. A systematic review of the effect of primary care-based service innovations on quality and patterns of referral to specialist secondary care *British Journal of General Practice* 2003; **53**: 878–84.

7. O'Donnell CA. Variations in GP referral rates: what can we learn from it? *Family Practice* 2000; **17**: 462–71.

8. Tuckett D, Boulton M, Olson C. *Meetings between Experts* London: Routledge, 1985.

CHAPTER 7

Medics are from Mercury and patients are from Pluto

Managers must be from Mars, then.   (Apologies to John Gray)

A consultation might be unsuccessful or uncomfortable for many reasons but we all acknowledge that a failure of communication is commonly part of this. There is a lack of clarity by GPs as to whose responsibility that failure might be and perhaps a reluctance to look at their part in this.

This chapter tries to encourage doctors to view basic communication skills as needing regular thinking about as often as, say, hypertension guidelines with some examples of what can be done. But we also look at the need for a doctor-defined boundary of care, which allows us to be good communicators within limits. Acknowledging that we cannot meet all expectations we start to look at being comfortable and certain in what we can do.

The sense that there is a large cultural, not to say astronomical, gulf between doctors and their patients is ever present, endlessly baffling both. We strive for patient-centredness though we pay for it with greater perceived stress, even if a positive I-can-help-you attitude correlates well with patient satisfaction.[1] Perhaps what we seek would be patients who are capable of being doctor-centred – what a fine idea! They would be considerate of our feelings and evaluate our situations in the wider psycho-social context, supporting us with higher status and perhaps pay; they would use our time judiciously and of course ask our views on what seems to be the best option before stating theirs. The doctor-centred patient might have an awareness of a GP's educational level and pitch his or her vocabulary effectively and might join participation groups and supportive organisations to make life a bit more comfortable for the clinical staff.

Hang on though. The patients already have some awareness of our circumstances and generally regard us as respectable individuals, they tend to be supportive of medical institutions and plans, and there is a strong movement from patients to involve themselves in medical education. Perhaps then patients are more doctor-centred than we give them credit for.

But there is still this gulf of apparent misunderstanding that the GP has a duty to try to overcome, even when 'fault' lies with the patient. Does this mean that doctors must always make the bridge and if they fail it is a sign of incompetence on their part? Clearly no, as sometimes patients will either consciously or unconsciously try to control the consultation in a way that is ultimately to their detriment. They might withhold information, be verbally aggressive or intimidating, or simply have no idea what the doctor's role is (an educational or cross-cultural problem perhaps). But our duty is clearly to try hard to meet patients more than half way, which means sometimes the patient seems to be not very helpful at all. Stress might be defined as three of those in a row.

A perilous stage in our history

History taking by GPs, emphasised as the core of the job, seems to make them nervous. Yet how many of us include updating our skills in this field as part of our Personal Development Plans (PDPs)? We leave it to the registrars to be the only ones interested in video analysis, and that is primarily in order to pass exams and assessments. The idea of the next section is to show that thinking about consulting styles need not be threatening and is potentially most enlightening, even for experienced doctors set in our ways.

The hardest aspect to the initial phase of history taking by doctors and nurses seems to be shutting up. After the initial greetings and hellos – building rapport – many doctors, not just the inexperienced, set the ball rolling with an open question but then keep going with a barrage of directed ones. To be effective, clinicians only have to be quiet, bar grunts and nods, for 60 to 90 seconds to get some priceless nuggets of information and an idea of where it is all going to head. That is the time needed to read a page of this book, so here is a one-page box, which would take that long to read if it had words in. Try looking at the page for that long; some intrusive thoughts will appear. But the idea is to listen to the page not read it; this is very hard and most of us GPs need regular training. Here goes:

(patient is being very vague)

(must ask…)
(wish they'd get on with it)

(must try to concentrate on them and not that distant phone, the clock or my bladder)

(ah, that sounds interesting)

(someone else's phone ringing)

(that bit needs some more detail)

> If you got to this point almost immediately you might be in danger of asking closed questions too early. Consider going back to the beginning.

The patient has by now poured out all of his or her muddled thoughts and ideas, some or much of which are not at all relevant to the medical aspects of his or her story. The GP needs quite a bit of Rapid Access Memory (RAM) to hold it all in, because it is necessary to make it tidy before it gets filed on the relatively hard drive of the brain. Therefore the GP has to pick up some of the bits and ask about them more, or carefully ask if there are any other bits not yet covered, and all the time being conscious that asking a closed question will get a closed answer and waste time asking it again, in a different way, in a moment. The experienced history taker does not try to direct the patient into giving the story in a tidy manner, and knows that 20 seconds spent trying to coax the patient towards greater clarity by using narrow, closed questions can mean a minute spent listening to repeated stuff he or she already knows. So the GP shuts up, and actually gets to the point more quickly. Studies of patient–doctor communications have shown that clinicians who adopt the open listening approach, at least at first, do not have longer consultations, but they do have more effective ones.[2]

The unconfident GP does not feel he or she can trust the patient to bring up the good stuff along with the rest, and is overly conscious of time. Videos of anxious consulters show them sitting earnestly forwards, perhaps making eye contact too strongly, interjecting repeatedly or asking questions in batches of two or three as they race to the diagnosis and then direct the cure or at least the plan of action. Fortunately patients are resilient and once interrupted many will, like the video-tape itself, automatically rewind and start again. The hurried clinician is flustered by such poor use of his or her precious time.

The garrulous

It is easy to generalise and clearly sometimes special circumstances mean the GP has to be less patient-centred. To unravel the useful strands of history from the truly garrulous might be one example, where sometimes the doctor has to, preferably non-verbally, get the patient to shut up. An increasing use of the hands angled in the way that a duck uses its feet as air-brakes is effective, finally *in extremis* ending in the hands actually being between the faces of patient and GP. Verbosity might itself be a sign of the mental state of the patient and feeding the observation back might be revealing – 'You seem rather nervous about this....'

Another fraught situation is the patient heavily under the influence of alcohol or drugs, the former maudlin and self-absorbed bores presenting to most doctors in most surgeries (and hospital departments) at times. The value to be gained from listening in this situation has to be measured against the time it might take and the outcome it might generate, but being truly patient-centred is not, perhaps, a realistic approach. Considering telling the patient to go away might be more so. Phone the Samaritans, contact a friend, whatever, but the GP has little to offer the truly drunk, except to make an arrangement to see them when they are sober.

Parents and children

To work with children and not have your own must be especially difficult. Parenthood allows a certain disinhibition, which is amusing and alarming to non-parents. For instance, young-adult non-parents look on appalled as experienced mums and dads try to decide if a nappy needs changing. In the world of nappy advertising this is done with decorum and delicacy, but in real life parents learn to thrust their nose heartily and deeply into the baby's heavily padded bottom and snort. Similarly the real-life mum and dad have a whole lot more tricks than a grin and a coo when communicating calm to a fractious baby, and these are a challenge to the unconfident, non-parent doctor. This is especially so when the infant patient might have good reason to be fractious and cross, as will usually be the case. Yet the right level of communication of calm can not only keep the volume down, but it can also be essential to the infant's care, such as when the child has a nasty and distressing wheeze.

The techniques for getting a child to relax are going to depend on getting the parent (or carer, but let's stick to parent) to feel calm first, which in turn means ways of getting them to feel reassured. The next chapter discusses this more fully. If the child has reached the age when this is an issue as well, then clearly their fears need addressing too. But the younger infant might need to see the GP as a benign and helpful adult, and it is only by practice that the different ways of winning over a child can be tried out. The non-parent will need to give him or herself permission to be silly to do this, with funny noises, pulled faces and odd playthings. Rather obviously all GPs need to know the name of their patient and his or her age, and be able to deduce or ask about his or her capabilities. They should wear suitable clothing so the consequence of cuddling and confidently holding a child who is prone to puking do not lead to a sort of arm's length revulsion. They need to know how to hold children aged up to perhaps a year, because there is much information to be gained from that, and the child and parent will enjoy it. However, examining the child on a parent's lap, which might feel a bit intimate and awkward, will often be the only way for older children. At the risk of being repetitive no clinician should feel this is all instinctive; it is learnt behaviour and they might, if they find they are alarmed by children, need to explore ways of getting past that.

The unfamiliar

In a society with many cultures the ideal GP would have a profound understanding of the cultures with whom he or she dealt. This is much more than language, as anyone who has had American, Scandinavian or medically qualified patients will testify. We can talk comfortably in English with these groups (unlike, say, with Middle Eastern asylum seekers or Polish migrant workers) yet the communication difficulties are profound because of our underlying differences in health beliefs, expectations and understanding of the role of a GP. There are pleasures to be had from doing some cross-cultural work and doctors have to read and learn their material from elsewhere, but they need to do it well. But common to all cross-cultural consultations will be the problem of establishing the story and the patient's expectations. Some cultures will have a very different view of the clinician's role and abilities, either higher or lower than the GP has of him or herself. Some might be very diffident about voicing this too.

Communication skills training forms a centrepiece of the UK undergraduate medical curriculum now, so there is an acceptance by younger UK-trained people that they need to work at this and not adopt what might be seen as instinctive or common-sense attitudes to dealing with patients. It is more difficult than that. The cultures from which the clinicians themselves come to work in the NHS are excitingly varied but present particular challenges to their practice. Doctors trained in South Asia or Europe, and nurses from Africa and the Caribbean, are surely working in every trust and Primary Care Organisation (PCO). But those GPs who trained overseas and those who trained in the UK some time ago are sensitive, and might feel threatened if anyone suggests that a particular medical encounter would have had a better outcome if the doctor was a more successful communicator. Clinicians not trained or used to the idea of training in communication skills are frequently shy of venturing into this area – it is much easier to fill one's Continuing Personal Development (CPD) time with learning about advances in asthma care, surgical technique or therapeutics. To have one's communication style criticised when one views it as part of one's inner being, as integral as the ability to do exams, remember numbers or learn the piano, is like being told one has a personality disorder. It feels not only pejorative, but also hopeless. This makes it very difficult for those in charge of CPD to advise on the area. Yet these skills are learnt ones, and need upgrading in time, and if we wish to be liked by our patients then it is by these means they judge us.

Admitting the problem

The elderly Sikh man attended me in the emergency primary care surgery late one night with the combined family acting as a sort of team interpreter. He had an alarming story of chest pain, sweating, nausea, dizziness. The diabetes from which he suffered came to light when the carrier bag of his medication was emptied on to the bed. Although he had no chest signs he did not look well and a myocardial infarction (MI) seemed a strong possibility. Without waiting for an opinion from him I said this and suggested to the family that we should get him to the hospital immediately.

Consternation. Could I not do something else?

What were you thinking of?

We don't know, you're the doctor.

I think he needs to be admitted. Irked tone creeping into my voice. The conversation dashed around this circle a few times.

We made no progress. Then I remembered my colleague on duty with me was originally from the Punjab and might communicate the urgency of the problem more effectively. Fetching her, I explained the problem. She is not a fan of new ideas like patient-centredness and sharing options. Indeed the body language she adopted, standing over the old man, arms folded, eyes pinned on him rather coldly, fell into my stereotyped view of her. Obviously I grasped none of the verbal exchange. Within a few minutes she had obtained a completely different history and reached a diagnosis of recurrent alcohol-induced gastritis. This had not occurred to me. She agreed a plan with the family, told him off in a way that I can only guess will have shaken him into lifelong sobriety, and he went home.

What's he doing here?

To help the discussion on the value of learning about better communication, I wish to rise to the challenge of making a sore throat interesting. This presentation is seen as the bore of primary care, our speciality, but all jobs have a mundane and repetitive side, and primary care no more than any other. The analogy with pretty well any other branch of medicine is clear. This list is a distillation of why the symptom is frustrating to GPs. Although I am looking at sore throats, it could apply to dyspepsia, haemorrhoids, vaginal discharges, insomnia, backache, atypical chest pains, constipated children, intractable 'depression' and much more.

- The condition is boring because it is rarely curable, and often self-limiting so GPs have better things they can be doing to increase the sum total of human happiness than spending time on this.

- Patients have access to home remedies and reasonable advice, and don't take them.

- Patients often present with remarkably minor signs.

- Primary care clinicians are inconsistent in their management of the problem.

- Research evidence is voluminous but doesn't seem to move us on very far.

- Patients seem to think that we can do more than we can, and that if we do not seem to give a treatment it is because of a moral judgement that they do not deserve to be relieved of their agony.[3]

But life is more complicated because we know, and patients probably know, that sometimes the sore throat is more medically exciting. Perhaps it is:

- a serious disease, like a tumour

- a treatable condition like a peritonsillar abscess, or a foreign body

- iatrogenic like steroid-induced candidiasis

- part of a wider condition like glandular fever.

So part of us knows that the patient has a legitimate view in getting the symptom checked out. The problem is numbers from the GP point of view, in that for the entire list above there are 99 additional minor virus infections. We will assume that the above conditions are seen as quite challenging and interesting problems that the doctor is pleased to be of assistance with. (If this is not the case, then career guidance is more likely to be of use than this book.). So from here on we are discussing the minor cases of sore throat and trying to nurture some professional enthusiasm about them.

The trick is to find out why the patient came. The answer is not, as many GPs would assert, always to get antibiotics, and the first danger is to assume that to be the agenda or even to assume we know anything about why they came.

The history needs to include a brief canter around the patient's life. His or her job, responsibilities, family. It needs to include not only a (again, brief) history of the complaint, i.e. previous episodes and how they were managed, but also that of the family. The story needs to include what it is the patient is unable to do, apart from swallowing comfortably, that they would wish to as a result of the symptom – work, sport, go to a party, take an exam, visit grandma in hospital or fly on holiday. Here lie some juicy points of interest, in which the patient becomes a person with complex family influences and a set of possibly erroneous health beliefs. The patient's expectations, if they have not emerged already, might need teasing out, and this is a task as delicate as microsurgery. They might not know them, they might be reticent (embarrassed, or intimidated) and it might not be their expectations that are important but those of someone at home. The precise fears of the patients need defining, such as febrile fits, gagging, pneumonia or might be a fear of being asked to swallow tablets. Again, this is communication microsurgery.

The GP needs to observe who else is in the room, because adult patients attending with a relative are communicating something and the game is to find out what. The relative might be a real nag, or worrier, and indeed is the sicker person in a way – but he or she might be exasperated by the patient too. The relative's presence might create confidentiality problems if an issue arises around a different disease the patient has, and the socially delicate task of evicting someone from the room is a considerable skill.

And having done all this in short shrift, the confident GP will get nowhere until not only has he or she got a handle on the patient or parent's expectations but also their willingness to negotiate, and reason. There might be a long list of issues the doctor has to sort out here:

- legitimising the attendance and the symptoms, even while trying to prevent future ones for this problem – 'I can see it is sore…'

- explaining the likely course of the condition, the powerlessness of medical science to alter it, and the pros and cons of different ways of relieving symptoms

- listening to the response and going through it again

- discussing up front the patient's expectations of treatment, and prescribing analgesia if agreed

- discussing the secondary issues of time off from work, or anything else, and what might be 'reasonable' and issuing permissive notes if agreed

- discussing any long-term issues, like tonsillectomy and how medical science has turned away from this but we can always hope

- admitting it could all go wrong and that, if it does, explain how to spot that and when the patient would need to return or seek help

- maintaining a trusting relationship throughout

- trying to give the patient confidence to self-care next time, ideally by somehow checking his or her understanding of all of the above.

There might be a judgement to be made about how much can actually be covered, but most of it will need to be there and then.

The secondary issues such as time off school and work need skill and judgement if the GP is going to challenge the patient. A week off might seem a lot for the symptoms as reported and there might be reasons to do with work rather than the sore throat that need to be understood. Then again many of these patients are young adults with an illness that a parent used to take care of, and they need guidance or their employer or college will take the view they are taking too much sick leave and their career or job be threatened. To cover this area sympathetically is hard and there is an ethical argument that GPs must aim to be the patient's advocate, not mentor, and they should work on behalf of the patient before employer or society. But the ethics are complex and the confident clinician strives for clarity on the issue.

Finally, exhausted, the clinician has to control the use of time and yet the patient has to feel he or she is in charge.[4]

To do this successfully without training and by instinct alone is implausible. The simplest way of rising to this challenge is to video the process and score it – a number of templates and systems are available (via your educational adviser).

Looked at in detail, then the case is hardly uninteresting. Until one has four cases in a row of course.

The boundary

- From time to time a controversy arises about smoking and refusing surgical treatment. Some doctors argue that because the results of surgery such as, say arthroplasty, are worse in smokers (more infections and joint failures) they should be denied it, as if the doctor were personally responsible for the infection.[5]

- In mid-2003 Ian Huntley, an inmate awaiting trial for the murder of two children, which he denied but for which he was later convicted, was on amitriptyline. He carefully hoarded them as they were issued and over some weeks had a sufficient number to take a major and near-fatal overdose, despite being very closely supervised in the prison. The furore and subsequent inquiry focused on the systems within the prison and what went wrong; the fault was assumed to be in there.

- I looked after a care worker who was suspended for assaulting a patient with severe learning difficulties in a residential home. But the patient, an adolescent boy, was sexually assaulting another resident who was sitting on the toilet, by groping her with his hand. He would not stop and pull away; so the carer smacked him on his bottom, which startled him into acknowledgment and allowed her and her assistant to pull him away from the victim safely.

These incidents illustrate a boundary between the patient's responsibilities and the clinician's or carer's. The boundary gets crossed more easily when it is indistinct and ideally society would clarify it for us all. However, it is far more in the interests of one party, the carers and doctors, than the patients to define it, and so clinicians should feel they have a right to do so. In other words, doctors need a line, an edge to their responsibilities in order to function. No one else will draw it, so we should. We are reasonable and helpful professionals, and will draw the line generously. This concept of a boundary seems to separate the unconfident from the confident decision maker more than almost any other.

The government has been helpful in discussing and drawing a line around violence; there is theoretically no tolerance of it and if the patient's care is compromised as a result of his or her violent behaviour, or the significant threat of it, then that is the consequence of his or her action. Violence against staff in NHS 'front-line' care has always happened and staff have always known and taken that risk, but the risk to them is greater if they felt they would be criticised for not dealing with the patient as they would any other. Yet the situation is not simple because the majority of patients who attack doctors and nurses are confused, have a mental health problem, or have (in mitigation) a grievance. Muggers, robbers and mindlessly violent youths are a problem but not the biggest one. The first two categories of patient are not ones where the patient can be said to have responsibility, or at least not full responsibility. So 'zero tolerance' is not always appropriate. Even in situations involving an aggrieved patient or relative where there is no excuse for violence and should be no tolerance of it, somewhere along the line many of these incidents could have been handled better. There are some simple and effective techniques for coping with threatening situations, which GPs and doctors who deal with them have to try – but if the problem is still not defused then sensible GPs retreat and call for physical back-up. They feel resigned, and content to prioritise their right not to be injured above the patient's right to privacy, confidentiality and ideal care. In other words, in a physically threatening situation most GPs seem clear in their minds where the line of responsibility is. Then the doctor needs a sense that after he or she has done everything reasonable short of being a hero, responsibility for dealing with the threatened or actual violence passes beyond his or her boundary and into someone else's – the patient's, usually – and the clinician has not failed.

So the lines drawn by well-intentioned authorities still need clarifying and justifying by the person standing nearest to them.

There is unsurprising evidence that threats to clinician autonomy, such as threatening to get a second opinion, alter the doctor's behaviour to do as the patient demands even against the doctor's clinical judgement.[6] Here GPs are much more uncertain of themselves.

GPs will frequently encounter self-harming behaviour. The extreme end of the scale is the dramatic overdosing such as described above, or the threat to jump from a building, and most of us see few of those. But more minor self-harm, such as superficial wrist slashing, is perhaps more akin to bulimia or binge drinking, in that at a moment of crisis or stress as defined by the patient he or she gets some relief by abusing his or her body in this way. These are commoner, and wash up in all surgeries periodically. Then there is: dermatitis artefacta, where patients pick at their skin, creating a patchwork of sores and pustules; drug and substance abuse that has gone beyond the reasoning of stress and into pure hedonism; promiscuity in an age of lethal sexually transmitted diseases (STDs); and, worst of all, smoking.

Patients whose self-harming behaviour is confined to smoking are treated with some sympathy and understanding by the medical profession, few of whom enjoy a cigarette, but if a patient fails to stop smoking despite all the advice and support offered, then all doctors seem to feel comfortable with the idea that the patient has made a choice and is responsible for that. The court cases in which the cigarette companies are made to stand trial for the harmful consequences of the addictive properties of their product are based on alleged misinformation from decades ago and do not affect the general view that this is now a personal responsibility issue. Similarly, GPs feel a responsibility to educate the sexually active in the risks of STDs and a responsibility to provide the best and most accessible treatment, but I see no evidence that GPs see themselves as personally responsible for the current frightening rise in cases of Chlamydia. But if a patient repeatedly takes small overdoses or rips his or her gullet vomiting after a dinner of a kilo of chocolate and ice cream, then there seems some uncertainty. It feels as if this problem lies on our side of the line of responsibility; we should do more. And so if any greater consequence arises from the behaviour it feels, in part, to be the doctor's fault. Indeed, here the GP must take different responsibilities than with, say, our self-harming smoker because current wisdom categorises this behaviour as a possible sign of mental illness. As identifying mental illness is not always easy, primary care clinicians feel uncertain and fear they are 'missing' something – it's a worry.

The threat from patients to self-harm is to be taken seriously, obviously, but acceding to demands for whatever the patient wants, such as a lot of time, must be considered with only very great care. Yet justifying to themselves a refusal to do as demanded, the clinicians are in danger of labelling the patient as an attention-seeking malingerer. That way lies trouble for everyone. However, confident GPs need to:

- avoid the word 'fault' and banish it from their thinking as a destructive influence

91

- know their own limitations, and assess the risk of such patients only if they know how (but it is not too difficult)

- take a history and listen as you would with any other patient

- legitimise the problem ('I can see you need help') and then

- find out their expectations ('How do you feel I can help?')

- negotiate with the patient the line of responsibility ('I would like to listen and hear how things are at home, though I can't change x, y and z'). With a smoker one would comfortably agree openly about the consequences of what he or she is doing ('I think your COPD will become worse if you keep smoking and we won't be able to help much'). Likewise, with these patients it might be necessary to point out you cannot stop them bingeing, and they will need to work with the professionals to crack this addictive behavioural response. Until they can agree to the pain and effort of change, and they might not be capable of that, then the goal is limited to harm minimisation and it will not always be possible even to do that

- avoid re-negotiating and be firm with the limits of their time and possibilities

- be comfortable, be sad, weep for the patient, but don't feel it is your responsibility when the patient hurts.

The myth of shared care and the rise of guidelines

This section on expectations and lines of responsibility needs to include a discussion of these other systems of delivering packages of care, which are becoming more prevalent and practically imposed.

Shared care started life in the antenatal clinic when women would alternate between the doctor and midwife, or the GP and hospital, for their basic checks as the pregnancy inched on. It works to a point in that once the patients were accepted as the owners of their care and, in particular of their notes, then the various clinicians could see exactly what was being done in the other clinic and monitor and contribute to the patient's care. Some things are better done in hospital, like scans, and others in the community, like blood pressure checks. But in the end the big decisions are still between the chief, usually the obstetrician, and sometimes the patient, and not a team consideration.

This is good, because these are the people most qualified to make those decisions. But it is not shared responsibility.

Diabetic care has never managed to reach the same level of organisation, a wide variation appearing to exist between districts and an even wider variation between primary care teams in any one area. This means that the secondary care teams have to deliver a variable level of care depending on the level of enthusiasm of the local primary care teams. So the tendency is to play safe and head for delegated care rather than shared care – a missive from the centre saying please see this diabetic in three months and check his or her pulses and let us know, or whatever. The parallel with the patient encounters is clear – with some patients it is easier to agree where the line of responsibility is than with others, and there is a tendency in all relationships for the more senior party to impose his or her view anyway.

Anxiety about patchy performance from primary care, rarely spoken by the courteous secondary sector, contributes to another 'shared' care phenomenon: the hospital-based community nurse. The motivation behind these services is manifold and, apart from the above worry, include:

- saving beds, managing more poorly people at home

- not over-burdening the primary care team

- offering more support to the recently ill

- doing technical things at home that never used to be done outside hospital.

The variety of hospital-at-home services, in paediatrics, medicine, palliative care and urology, to name a few, expands all the time and it is not fashionable to question this. But apart from the mathematics – such services are tiny compared with the primary healthcare teams (PHCTs) and will only ever look after a tiny number of people – as ever the lines of responsibility are unclear or in the wrong place. These services have as a characteristic the right of re-admission back into the hospital, because the patient has never really left it and the result is that this is exactly what happens. But the unconfident secondary sector is not always the best judge of the need for admission, and the patient might sometimes have been better discharged to an effective PHCT, if there is one. The line of trust is not strong enough.

The primary care responsibility is to achieve clarity then of who does and can do what, the co-ordinator role rather than clinician. We need to have a good local knowledge of the secondary care sector, its resources and capabilities. Communications addressed as 'Dear colleague', as they now are, will not improve this.

Asking patients a favour and the balance of power

Very many GPs and PHCTs are involved in teaching, at some level, of entrants to the profession or perhaps of graduates progressing within their speciality. Like the care of patients generally the education of doctors and GPs in particular is protocol driven with a menu and objectives, and measurable outcomes above and beyond merely passing exams and pleasing the right people. So the curriculum is closely defined by the various authorities, and through their various inspection systems the authorities check on the educators, and that the learners have the full experience they need to become competent doctors and then GPs. There is leeway of course, and all teaching environments have strengths and weaknesses, but the idea is more consistent and effective education. So one can trust that the GP trained in Glasgow can objectively demonstrate sufficient experience to practise in Kent. This is important but puts great onus on the education system, and one by-product of this is that teacher-doctors, to make sure the learners see what they need to see, are asking favours from patients perhaps more than ever.

It is a challenging and stressful business asking patients to spare some time and effort to be used for education – for the net good of us all – rather than their own good. That there might even be harm to the patient has to be acknowledged, i.e. a patient might need to undergo a procedure, have a painful joint examined or have a sexual history taken, and it is the learner's first effort at it. To ask that patient explicitly is difficult for the teacher and many consent protocols are drawn up to meet the ethical challenge involved. However, more commonly in primary care the patient is not so much taking a personal risk, but being asked to give a routine history and perhaps be examined. Fortunately there is ample altruism out there, or perhaps a lot of bored patients, and sufficient recruitment for the educators' purpose can be achieved.

The price is the alteration in the doctor–patient relationship. At the moment of the request the normal power held by the clinician is sidelined and the control, assuming the matter is being approached sensitively, is in the patient's hands. The teacher-doctor is briefly in unfamiliar territory; the patient might exercise his or her power and decline, and one trusts that is the end of the matter. If the patient agrees to grant the favour, though, the matter will often hang there in future encounters. So although the issue might be a fairly small one for the GP, it will be recalled, perhaps unspoken, at his or her next, clinical, encounter with the patient. There sometimes develops a feeling of a favour not paid back – the patient might want a little extra time, or something sorted that is a little above and beyond normal practice for the GP, and some will ask for it openly. The doctor has a momentary dilemma that is uncomfortable. More usually, he or she will feel an obligation to offer before being asked, or at least appear to him or herself to make the extra effort for the pliant patient who has been so helpful previously. Whatever happens the doctor–patient relationship is altered, and it takes a confident clinician to either re-establish the rules and boundaries or accept the new ones.

Conclusion

This chapter has covered in an absurdly short time some issues of communication and relationships with patients that can contribute to a GP's failure of confidence to make a reasonable decision from the consultation. To recap:

- communication skills are learnt and not innate
- there are good ways of learning them but it takes some courage to admit that one needs specific action. The rewards in terms of better consultations are well worth it

- primary care clinicians need a sense of boundary that must ultimately come from their own sense of reasonableness, because no one else will define it clearly

- if a patient has every opportunity to get help and state what he or she needs, and there is no reasonable barrier to this, then the responsibility is the patient's, not the doctor's, to see that such help is obtained

- boundaries between clinicians need to be respectful, and explicit, or there is danger. GPs especially have to know exactly what other clinicians do

- the conflict between the needs of society to have educated professionals and the autonomy of patients in negotiating who they have caring for them, and what their relationship is like with these professionals, is difficult. The doctor in an educator role must understand this to some depth, therefore, to remain confident of his or her role.

References

1. Howie J, Hopton J. Attitudes to care, the organisation of work and stress amongst GPs *British Journal of General Practice* 1992; **42**: 181–5.

2. Silverman J, Kurtz S, Draper S. *Skills for Communicating with Patients* (second edn) Abingdon: Radcliffe Publishing, 2004.

3. MacFarlane J, Holmes W, Macfarlane R, *et al*. The influence of patient expectation on antibiotic management of acute lower respiratory infection in general practice: questionnaire study *British Medical Journal* 1997; **315**: 1211–14.

4. Williams S, Weinman J, Dale J. Doctor–patient communications and patient satisfaction *Family Practice* 1998; **15**: 480–92.

5. Petere MJ. Should smokers be refused surgery? *British Medical Journal* 2007; **334**: 20–1.

6. Kristiansen I, Forde OH, Aasland O, *et al*. Threats from patients and their effects on medical decision making: a cross sectional randomised trial *Lancet* 2001; **357**: 1258–61.

I don't know what it is but I don't think it's meningitis

The crux of handling uncertainty in a consultation is getting across this concept to someone who was hoping for something better. This specific area is not covered in the standard communication textbooks. It is more than just giving information over and expecting the patient to grasp it. We are passing responsibility over in consultations where there is significant uncertainty and GPs have to do this skilfully to be effective and not swamped. This chapter is a practical discussion of these skills.

Who could be an optimist when his or her child is clearly dreadfully ill?

What is an optimist? The person who sunnily describes him or herself as an optimist is not someone who can see the bright side of all situations, but someone who sees the benign side of human nature before the malign one. They are able to focus on the pleasanter and more positive aspects of situations, perhaps. Actually we all have ways of coping with the worries of life, and experience suggests that the worst outcome in a crisis is also the least likely: the cock-up at work doesn't lead to a dismissal every time; the late teenager is not always a drugs and road traffic accident (RTA) victim; and the unpaid bill does not lead to homelessness. The optimist remembers this, even whilst aware that rare and disastrous outcomes do happen to others, because they are reported so fully, but appreciates that they really are rare. The pessimistic obverse to this view is the commonly held feeling amongst the elderly about their likelihood of being a victim of crime or parents' ideas about the chance of their children being hurt by strangers if left unsupervised to walk to school. The latter groups have arguably lost all sense of proportion, unable to agree that for nearly everyone, nearly all the time, life follows along an easier route and to adapt one's life to ease remote fears is to misjudge it.

But nothing levels humanity like health issues, personally threatening and overwhelming as they are. Neither those with a pessimistic temperament nor those with an optimistic one will find it easy to take a chance until they are feeling fully in charge, fully aware and confident in their advisers. Taking a chance in this context means coping with an uncertainty: coping with the responsibility of their own or someone else's ill health. All clinicians, especially GPs, experience the ways patients are tested by the uncertainty of disease, and most of us are impressed. We see a range of controlling responses from the managerial type who needs masses of data, to the inarticulate who nods in apparent acceptance of whatever is said. And we see the full range of emotions expressed by the uncontrolled patient, from displaced anger perhaps at us, to tears or accusations, withdrawal or flat disbelief. Everyone wants some reassurance and the wise GP is placed to give some, if not as much as would be wished.

The ironic title to this chapter is a condensation of what we are trying to say to patients all the time, only it is prone to coming out as inept, inaccurate, offensive, risky and crass, or possibly all of these things. Our current diagnostic and treatment plans might be cutting-edge stuff when we know what is happening, almost as if it was easy. But this chapter is about discussing the approach to the patient whose fears, at least at this moment, are worse than reality. It is more complicated than it first seems.

Planned sickness

We all have Personal Development Plans (PDPs) and annual appraisals now, the latter including a reflective section on our own health.

Well perhaps we should all be ill occasionally as part of our personal learning and development plans. If it might be devised that in some sort of way we experienced illness, but not, one hopes, its final consequence, we would learn. This is more than an appreciation of what pain is like or how distressing the nausea or incontinence or disability can be, because such experiences remain personal to the patient even if they happen to have a professional qualification. To extrapolate a personal experience of back pain to all patients who have it would obviously be wrong. Although probably most clinicians should have a barium enema at some point, just to make sure they stick to proven indications....

But we do need to empathise with the patient's experience of uncertainty as he or she hopes that the clinician in charge brings good and timely news. Imagine waiting three months for your HIV antibody result, say, following a possible exposure to the virus. Or having not only a back pain of uncertain origin, perhaps with some weight loss, but also all the ponderous tests that are likely to follow from such a presentation. Some of us will have gone through this anxiety and sought reassurance that the clinical adviser, at least at first, could not give; a small comfort might be that it surely makes us better at the job.

The GP's agenda

The first job for the GP must be to know his or her stuff. There is no point in trying to tell a patient that there is no sign of meningitis if the doctor does not know what the signs are or how to find them. But even so we might well find ourselves with situations that have the following characteristics:

- it is not a 'textbook case' of anything, but has a number of features of a mild condition at an early stage. However, a severe condition has not been excluded, and cannot be at this moment

- there is an implicit or explicit fear of the severe condition

- the patient is at this moment reasonably well, albeit with some symptoms

- the cost of subscribing to a defence society has just gone up again.

'Not a textbook case of anything' must be the most common diagnosis in medicine, and is encountered everywhere (and not just in primary care). The doctor can go so far towards putting a label on it, but has a judgement to make about how far to go. Since the patients are all different, then the idea that we should know everything is not realistic. Many a time patients are odd, unusual or different – or we have not at first given due weight to the different strands in the story that could help. The GP has therefore to know his or her stuff and yet know when he or she doesn't know too. This is where the GP is tempted to try to appear confident, bluffing a little perhaps ('It must be a virus'), and kidding no one. In previous eras the doctor might give the condition some long Latin label that had no explanation but a good sound to it – notoriously the dermatologists went for this technique. But the modern GP might now open a textbook or website in front of the patient and discuss the situation openly, starting to explore the next steps. Discussing with patients their unique set of problems, choosing to look something up in their presence, works and it has been shown patients do not mind this – the authority of the written word even in our cynical age is great.[1]

The GP might advise that uncertainty at the consultation in question is not an acceptable endpoint, of course. So we will arrange to investigate even fairly minor post-menopausal bleeding, and work to exclude a treatable lethal condition of uterine cancer, and will not settle for the label 'post-menopausal bleeding ? cause'. In fact reassurance even at the initial outpatient clinic appointment will be limited, and the reader is referred to the considerable literature on Breaking Bad News.

But, continuing with the gynaecology theme, there are many causes of pelvic pain and the GP-gynaecologist knows some he or she can make a fairly confident diagnosis with, and some cases will ultimately be advised to proceed to laparoscopy, with its small but measurable risks. Again, if there is news, good or bad, then that is discussed.

And some will remain as 'pelvic pain ? cause' at least for a while. This is acceptable since of those some will spontaneously remit and save a lot of bother. The ones who were laparoscoped will be those with indications of severe disease, whose lives seem to be affected a lot, and/or who make the most noise. The latter group are ones for whom the reassurance to date has been either ineffective or is unacceptable because they are intolerant of uncertainty. Of course serious reassurance has not even been tried in some.

The true reassurance phase of the consultation – which might well be the latter part of a series of encounters over time rather than a single encounter – has to be prepared for. We are all advised that it is essential to be prepared with time and information when giving bad news; actually, giving good news (or an absence of bad news) might take a similar time. The doctor has concluded that it might be best at this point to adopt a wait-and-see strategy – masterly inactivity as it used to be called. The GP will have to be sure of him or herself and negotiate this as far as possible with the patient. If the GP is not sure if further investigation is needed then this uncertainty comes across and a spell of systematic reassurance is not what is needed. I wish to discuss the situation where the GP is confident at this moment that monitoring/watching is the best plan by far. But GPs will find the scenario quickly unravels if they spend most of their precious time re-familiarising themselves with the medical records in the patient's presence. This is perceived as discourteous, and it is better to have a shorter consultation with a little preparation time than a longer one with a frustrated patient.

Checking the patient's agenda

Agreeing a summary with the patient is an effective start, because it proves how good the GP is at listening and gives a chance to make sure the emphasis is right. The first person who needs reassurance is the doctor him or herself, to be confident that all the pertinent facts have been duly weighted in his or her mind.

> 'So you have had this tummy pain for a week, mostly on the left side, and you were sick at the start of it and have had diarrhoea too. But you've kept fluids down more recently. You were fine until then and are generally healthy.'
>
> 'Yes, but I should tell you the diarrhoea was only a couple of times and it was five days ago.'
>
> 'So the main problem is the pain still. Ah....'

The GP, about to put this down to gastro-enteritis, albeit rather long lasting, now has to consider other options and might even have to start again.

So what is the problem?

And then it is time to ask the patient what he or she thinks the problem is. There is a range of answers you might get here, and it depends on the way the matter is put. As some of the responses are going to be a bit sharp one has to be a touch thick skinned here.

They might have a particular fear that they share with you. In fact this is often volunteered earlier in the history taking and needs to be carefully noted by the GP for use later. The fear might need confirming, because until the GP knows what is really on the patient's mind, and everything to do with it, then the reassurance will fail. Repeating it back might be helpful ('You said you worried about osteoporosis') and trigger more information and further insights for the clinician, such as the family history or his or her bedtime reading and internet addiction – which might be useful at best and put some colour into the narrative at worst.

They might rebut the question and say it is the GP's job to tell him or her; that's why the patient has come. This response will occur from time to time, however delicately the question is put. Creeping up to the point of the question, rather than baldy asking what he or she is worried about, is best. For example:

> 'I was wondering what might have been going through your mind when the pain came on.'

or

> 'I wonder if you could help me. I don't think for a moment there is any very serious condition going on here, but I might be able to explain better why I think that, if I know your thoughts too.'

99

If the patient is not known to the clinician the language he or she will choose to use will have to be judged on the doctor's early impression, and it will go wrong sometimes.

They might have a fear but are not prepared to say what it is. This group is the greatest challenge and there follows a little banter, with the GP trying to see if the patient is too embarrassed to say, because to do so would make the patient appear ignorant or presumptuous – or perhaps the patient cannot bring him or herself to mention the very core of his or her fright, be it AIDS, cancer or dementia. Sometimes the patient will need very gentle coaxing, with phrases like 'There must be something you are concerned about here…you've gone to the trouble of seeing me' or 'Please don't be afraid to tell me what is on your mind because it will help me discuss with you what we should do.'

It might be necessary to use leading questions as a last resort, to be used only when all else fails for fear of the patient misleading you. A permissive statement like 'Some patients worry that this is meningitis…I was wondering what you were thinking' can work. It can also make you think he or she was worried about meningitis when the patient thought he or she had a migraine (but doesn't want to stop the pill).

The time taken to do this is minimal with practice, and an exploration of the patient's health agenda can usually be done in under a couple of minutes – honestly. And is highly cost-effective in terms of time spent later.

Who is involved?

So far we have told the patient very little. We have got as far as we reasonably think we should with the patient; we want to move on and feel that waiting and seeing is going to be a reasonable option here. We know where the patient's fears lie.

The next step, a form of avoidance possibly but also crucial to the success of this process, is to ask who should be doing the reassuring. Should the primary care clinician who knows the patient best be the person to conduct this? Occasionally a consultant might need to be involved to add authority to the reassurance, but this can be counter-productive. Some thought will need to be given here. But the GP should see that he or she has the skill and respect to do this in most situations.

The next stage is deciding who needs reassurance. The stakeholders in the process, to use the current jargon, are:

- the patient
- the GP and team
- the GP's baggage
- the supporting and undermining systems for the patient
- the supporting and undermining systems for the GP and team.

And you thought there were only two people in the room! But all but the loneliest patients go home and discuss, perhaps in an edited form, what went on at the consultation. Likewise GPs, who do not of course get to go home, share worries and fears with trusted colleagues. The sense of what these third parties might say and think is crucial to the words used by the doctor in the next few minutes.

The GP's baggage

This is the theme of this book, in so far as there is one, and at the risk of repetition the confident GP is aware of a number of facts floating in the murky soup of uncertainty, such as:

- often you can't tell a patient that he or she doesn't have cancer, or heart disease or whatever, because you know that, although the checks are clear, checks are not a guarantee. But *you can say that nothing we have found suggests that he or she has these illnesses.* On a few occasions in a professional lifetime the patient will later prove to have a sinister diagnosis; you were not wrong, but not right either. You set up a safety net system to catch him or her. The experienced GP has a sense of the statistics of this, and does not permit undue influence from past events to get in the way of giving essentially good news

- we often tell patients that it is 'very difficult to diagnose meningitis in the earliest stage' – untrue. No. Wrong, wrong, wrong. It's not difficult; it is in fact impossible. To believe that something is merely 'very difficult' implies that it is nevertheless possible, and that one should strive even harder (more checks, more tests, cleverer doctors, surely something could be done?). But since the task proves *de facto* impossible, this just makes the GP feel perennially inadequate.

Strong GPs know within their field what is possible and what is impossible, and that occasional miracles are lucky breaks and no more. But they also keep up to date and know what within the 'possible' category is within their skill and power.

Behind the patient

So they might well have explained that they were fearful of cancer, TB, losing independence or quite possibly just of not getting better before their holiday in Spain. But in the case of primary care it is known that even before patients make an appointment they have discussed with family and perhaps friends whether to see the doctor or nurse at all. And an encounter with the secondary sector might have been the referrer's idea, although not necessarily; patients request referrals or self-present via A&E to get into the system. Either way, the influence of relatives who are not with the patient might well be strong and so our attempt at reassurance, which we plan to undertake, might fall flat, because it is not the patient who is worried. This might not be mentioned!

The patient might well also have some issues with previous medical encounters that lead to certain behaviours and expectations, whether the experience was positive or negative. So if our nurse practitioner is trying to calm a patient with a recurrent sore throat and is unaware that the patient's niece had something similar and it turned into glandular fever, and the doctor never mind the nurse didn't spot it, and she had a year off college because of it, then paracetamol-soaked platitudes are not going to reassure him or her. The patient might not have volunteered that glandular fever was his or her concern because of knowing that for some reason it is not the diagnosis in his or her case, but might have heard that no sore throat can be treated until a blood test is done, or a swab taken. If the patient is upfront it is easy to sort out: if not then, in the end, there is only so much the GP or primary care clinician can be expected to deduce.

Behind the GP

There is a lot of experience and wisdom, but not enough distillation of it. Chapter 6 explores further the necessity of discarding difficult cases, so we can stick with our evidence-based pathways for the moment.

Defensive medicine is the antithesis of the reassurance consultation, given that what we are trying to achieve with the patient is a comfortable agreement to accept a 'safe' risk.[2] Lawyers seem to find risk to be an unacceptable concept with the great lengths they go to, to anticipate risks and provide for them in impenetrable contracts and deals. Doctors and nurses receive ample guidance from the lawyers who might have to represent them on avoiding risks and to be fair much of their advice is obvious and sound, like keeping clear and legible notes. But such guidance nevertheless does seem to be written from an angle that is unfamiliar with the daily life of the GP, if only from time pressures. There is a continuous sense that if something has gone wrong then it might have been avoided by spending a little extra time doing (insert defensive medicine activity here), as if we all had a little extra time for each patient but used it for a coffee break.

Taking the blame

Politicians are not allowed to take risks either. They are castigated for not making life utterly safe, the daily moans in the media that this or that event shows that someone must have been responsible somewhere. Sometimes the media is right, of course, and there is an issue of judgement or competence by an individual. Often the result, though, of getting a single issue out of proportion will be some badly misjudged legislation like the infamous Dangerous Dogs Act or over-the-top fire regulations.

The 'shouldn't you have known better' brickbat hurled by a journalist at a leader of some sort has painful echoes for any doctor who has been involved in a complaint around a rare or exceptional case. An event is distilled by a journalist to a tidy, inadequate snippet describing some failure, implying an individual (or group or whole profession) is at fault for their ignorance. The defence of the politician might be to deflect the blame but do something to avoid the problem in the future like pass a law. The GP, however, who can see the bigger picture of a great deal of effective work under threat from new regulation, does not see that, and might privately challenge the premise that the single event is symptomatic of a common fault. But rarely feels confident in saying so. Thus the GP is hauled up for not referring all his wet-nosed patients to a (mythical) allergy clinic and his or her nurse is held to account for following rigid and slow (but safe and well-audited) protocols.

Journalists, like refuse collectors, are a vital part of our society but refuse gives a very limited view of what is really going on in the house. The doctor has to learn to identify good evidence-based journalism from the rubbish and be influenced appropriately. The problem of course is that quite a lot of rubbish is well written.

GPs have to be aware that leadership by lawyers and politicians is thus hampered by the system, and to give undue weight to such risk-averse professions will sap their confidence and be unfair to their patients.

So the primary care clinician is not likely to have a comfortable sense of understanding, daily support from the Secretary of State or even his or her lawyer. The support needed to work well with the patient on managing a touch of uncertainty will come only from his or her own institution, mostly the clinician's peers. And of course if he or she perceives that this support won't materialise when it is needed, then the clinician will resort to a dull and expensive, rather isolated, life of playing safe. I contend that such an approach does not lead to better sleep.

Elsewhere I rattle on about respecting managers and colleagues. This is where their presence is needed, where the GP is being asked to be the messenger for the system which is telling the patient that, at this point, no further action is really needed because we expect everything to go well. Yet that messenger might feel he or she is also facing a fusillade of diktats and must-dos which imply that support is only available for those doctors who follow the rules precisely (whether such shots come from the Department of Health, the *Sun* or the *Today* programme). The diktats and must-dos might not really be that fierce and actually only be some ideas and advice, but the fear of complaints can dominate. The GP might then go into defensive medicine mode and we are all the poorer.

A journalist explains to a patient's parent that he or she doesn't know what it is but doesn't think it is meningitis...

'So how did you feel when you thought he had meningitis?'

'Well, I was worried, you know....'

'But you must have been very upset....'

'Well obviously it was on my mind, with the headache and fever and that....'

'Yes but we know it isn't meningitis now and I'm delighted to say he's going to be alright.'

'Are you sure? He looks poorly to me.'

'No, he'll be fine. Trust me.'

'Well what's wrong with him then?'

'I don't know, but I've been told he is fine.'

'What should I do?'

'Oh I should think paracetamol, fluids, the usual sort of thing.'

'Can I call you if there's a problem?'

'What?'

A lawyer explains to a patient's parent that he or she doesn't know what it is but doesn't think it is meningitis...

'Now I have looked at all the paperwork and your son, and then the paperwork again, and we think it is on the whole, at this moment, unlikely that, given the evidence we have to date (and this is provisional as we discussed earlier) and the limitations of the clinical skills which I and indeed all practitioners at this level are able to bring to bear on this circumstance, that is to say the level of skill and care one would normally expect from a clinician in these circumstances THAT the issue of meningitis is presently NOT in the forefront of the diagnostic possibilities pertaining to the case NOTWITHSTANDING that further developments, changes, deteriorations and acts of God might cause us to review the situation at the sole discretion of the responsible adult WHEREIN the above opinion will be rendered null and void, and no liability can be accepted on the part of the clinician, his employers or the secretary of state for health.'

'Eh?'

'Could you sign here?'

> ### A politician explains to a patient's parent that he or she doesn't know what it is but doesn't think it is meningitis...
>
> 'Now my dear I am delighted to be able to tell you that he does not have meningitis and I am assured by my officials that....'
>
> 'Well what does he have then?'
>
> 'Assured by my officials that everything possible will be done to find an answer to that very good question....'
>
> 'He looks pretty unwell to me. I'm very worried you know. It's easy for you....'
>
> 'Good question as I say. If I might answer, I think you have had a very worrying time and I do understand that, but he will be fine, I promise you, before you know it.'
>
> 'Are you going to see him tomorrow and check then?'
>
> 'I have a very important meeting tomorrow, unfortunately, but perhaps you could speak to one of my officials?'
>
> 'Get stuffed.'

The cynical and stereotyped vignettes in the boxes are there to remind us that, in the end, clinical explanations especially to the worried not-very-ill are best done by the GP. To take guidance from professions who are trained to look at life from a different angle would be wrong.

The denouement

Avoiding saying what you think

If there is a possibility of avoiding giving an opinion, then our sensible GP will consider that seriously. He or she knows that the worst thing would be to give a weak opinion, which leaves the patient with the sense that the situation is out of control and the clinician is not competent to sort it out, so they will have to cope somehow alone, as in the blunt title of this chapter.

But giving no opinion at all might suit some patients who are prepared to go down a logical pathway and weigh the personal facts themselves in order to form their own view and plan. Thus one might be in the situation of:

1. The patient has symptoms that are usually called non-cardiac chest pain or atypical chest pain or another synonym. He or she has some features reminiscent of the sort we were all told about in medical school to be typical for angina and some features that are not

2. The patient is worried it is a cardiac problem and has said so

3. The patient has some 'risk factors' and has undergone numerous tests short of angiography, which are all clear

4. The GP is not keen to progress to more tests because the history does not suggest it is warranted and the effect on the patient's lifestyle is mild

5. The doctor is under pressure to conserve resources and wants to discharge the patient. But he or she knows from experience that a bald statement that there is nothing wrong with his patient's heart is both ineffective (the patient will keep coming to the clinic if not buying the explanation) and possibly hazardous (the patient still has risk factors).

A strategy might be to get the patient to enlarge on why he or she thought the problem was cardiac, i.e. what features of the illness did the patient note that were particularly alarming. Then the patient might need to have each bit of his or her symptomatology acknowledged and, assuming we do not actually know the exact cause of the pains and so on, an explanation given as to why that symptom is not at all like a cardiac pain.

'These pains are pretty unpleasant at times but the fact that it is on the right and seems to affect your breathing makes it far from likely that it is heart trouble. Heart pain is not generally like that.'

or

'The sweatiness can indicate all sorts of things, and doesn't indicate the problem is one from the heart. It might be related to weight (ahem) or to nerves for instance.'

Still the wily GP has not given an opinion on the actual patient's case.

They might try asking 'If we agree this is not a heart problem, what do you feel it might be?'

Some patients will volunteer a far more plausible explanation, such as panic attacks or 'nerves'. Either the GP then accepts the patient's opinion and reinforces it with examples and explanations about what he or she thought was going on along the same lines, or the GP has to refute this one too. (The experienced GP finds that sometimes there is a temptation to accept an explanation of 'nerves' offered by a patient who feels he or she can go home and cope, in lieu of an organic possibility that the patient would rather not think about, but which has, unfortunately, occurred to the clinician.)

Nevertheless the overall aim is to get the patient to convince him or herself that this situation is not so bad. The patient perhaps needs to be allowed or even encouraged to go through a mental sequence starting with 'I have symptoms X, Y and Z, which mean I might be suffering from angina. I told my doctor who seemed to think I might be right and examined me and did various tests. But I am not sure if I can trust the doctor/examination/tests.'

The doctor might think the information the patient is short of is simply an alternative diagnosis. 'This is costochondritis; it is not serious, take these.' But the information the clinician actually needs to feed into the patient is 'X, Y and Z are not really symptoms amounting to angina' and then 'We cannot completely dispel this by an examination but the tests are helpful and they also show no sign of angina' plus 'We are good at finding bad news but not so good at explaining everyone's symptoms all the time.' Finally, 'This is quite a common situation, of which I have experience, and is usually best dealt with by symptomatic relief.'

If we can get the patient to decide and preferably say out loud that he or she can see it is not angina then that phase of the job is done. And we have avoided committing ourselves to a spurious diagnostic label, and probably educated the patient, who remains at risk we remember, about heart disease. The patient will either lose weight, stop smoking and take up jogging, or else he or she will know what to look out for in the future.

Saying what you think

Some reassurance situations might need our hero to take the view that he or she will have to commit, much as it is against his or her instinct. The patient above might not be able to offer an alternative or have the understanding and possibly mental equipment and training to do any deduction him or herself. And a child whose parents fear that their eczematous rash is a sign of meningitis will harass A&E until someone deals with it.

The commitment must therefore be convincing and not only to the patient, but also to the family back home who will want the explanation too, only this time from our anxious and possibly inarticulate patient. This is where 'I don't know what it is but I don't think it's meningitis' becomes 'Nothing here suggests meningitis as you understandably feared. I think it is a typical virus illness with some eczema and we should treat it as such for the moment.'

The commitment, to a possibly spurious diagnosis, can be necessary and is not to be ashamed of so long as there is a way out. If ever the message comes across as 'This is trivial eczema and a bit of a virus, and you should know better than to waste my time. Go and buy some treatment' then the lawyers will surely not be far away.

The consultation is not over yet

The clinician must double check that the patient, and the carer or whoever is the one needing reassurance and a sense of control, is happy with this.

Most medical scenarios like this, which involve a small but present risk of an unexpected downturn in the patient's health, warrant safety netting. It is tempting to provide the blanket statement of 'If you're worried then just get back in touch'.

This is an approach that clogs every surgery, children's ward and NHS Direct with people who are, well, worried – but not ill. This is not the modern GP's approach, who seeks to achieve the following for his or her patients:

- confidence that patients understand the current situation, including the small level of risk

- patients have a sense of what might happen next and are not fearful of it. They have therefore an understanding if not a control of the position

- patients feel the GP's explanations can be trusted

- patients will manage the same or similar symptoms on their own in the future at least for a while *even though they are worried.* They know what doctors and nurses can and cannot do.

What have I just told you?

The process of safety netting needs to start from knowing what the patient has understood of the explanation so far. This is really difficult to ask without sounding like the deputy head reprimanding a child for being distracted by the view from the window during the teacher's exquisite explanation of tectonic plate theory.

In practice non-verbal cues have to be used very sensitively to get a feel for whether the patient has understood what you've said. The attentive patient, who has nodded and smiled at the right moment, and displays an open body position, probably does not need a quiz. The one with the sceptical look, crossed limbs and narrowed eyes might have understood what was said but not bought it yet – we have not yet succeeded in engendering trust.

It's the one who looks uncertain, fretful, leaning forward and struggling inwardly who might not have understood the words the GP used, and it might be necessary to check:

'Can I just check you've understood what I am trying to put across?'

or

'I'm sorry if I am not being clear – could you repeat back to me what I said so I can see if I put it over properly?'

or

'How did that sound? Could you reassure me you know what is going on?'

Obviously if there emerges a misunderstanding then it needs correcting.

Engendering trust in the clinician

In all the literature about communicating risk, it is clear that the communication fails if the patient cannot trust the clinician.

Fortunately we start from a higher base of trust than almost anyone else, so unworthy motives are not so likely to be ascribed to us automatically. Unfortunately we saw that before the late Harold Shipman's trial his surviving patients signed a petition of trust and confidence in him, which was about as misplaced as it is possible to be. One gathers Shipman gained the patients' trust with a strongly paternalistic approach – I am the doctor, the responsibility is mine and this is what I shall do. Other high-profile medical disasters like Bristol show this characteristic too. A category of patient appreciates this manner. The temptation of the doctor to gain such patients' respect by taking full charge of the patients' health is strong, given that the boundary is then so clear and some clinicians actually believe they have the power to carry it through. But it is of course a myth, and a benefit of our more critical society is that the modern primary care doctor, working to support the patient but not take them over, is better understood. The individual GP must earn respect from each of his or her patients, one by one, rather than assuming it to be his or her right, and when they do so the GP's confidence, and effectiveness, rises.

This is not too difficult. After all, confident GPs are clear why they are doing the job and can justify it to themselves and their patients if called upon to do so; the motives are not pure saintliness but they do coincide with the patient's interests.

Returning to the reassurance consultation it is apparent that the clinician might have said the child with the symptoms of a viral illness, or the man with the muscular chest pain, or whatever, is not showing signs of anything alarming. The patient has to trust that this is so, and this is based on the GP's communication skills and the value the patient has placed in the knowledge the GP possesses. But in the individual case, which the patient knows is not a textbook case, he or she wants as a basis of trust that the doctor has made a reasonable judgement. The doctor knows this is based very largely on the history. I have discussed above the value of including feedback in the explanation of the patient's history to illustrate that his or her feared condition is very unlikely (e.g. saying to the atypical chest pain patient who worried regarding heart pain 'The pain you are getting is not the sort we find indicates heart trouble' – the patient is thereby one hopes enlightened). Yet we find such communication skills are not appreciated as much as we would like. The patient will often feel a trustworthy opinion is based more on the physical examination or tests.

Consider this.

Patients sometimes report on other doctors, usually consultants, whom they have seen admiringly, with phrases like 'He gave me a very good examination'. This is usually referring to quantity (time taken, how many clothes removed, how many systems examined) rather than quality (the patient will not as a rule assess the detailed value of a fundoscopy or rectal examination, merely that it happened). Said doctor's pronouncements then undoubtedly carry extra weight. Similarly a test carries more reassurance value if it is complex or appears to be so.

But the fact that patients are giving an account of this to you, the GP they are now seeing, suggests this reassurance might have been incomplete. This does not quite add up and it seems the patient felt the examination/tests were indeed good but somehow slightly short of convincing.

The specialist might have failed to explain what the examination was for, what it was showing and why. We cling to the mystique of a physical examination as a biblical laying on of hands, this skill that separates us from the lay patient, and perhaps to boost our self-esteem we like the illusion that it is somehow terribly clever. We know the value of the hands-on bit is more subtle than the mere pursuit of a diagnosis, including as it does further opportunity for history taking and understanding, and the empathic touch of one human for another in distress. This makes it an invaluable help to the patient. But we can use the belief in the primacy of physical signs to demonstrate our trustworthiness too, so long as we are confident enough in ourselves to stop pretending that physical examination is always difficult, too clever for lay folk to grasp.

The reader will note that the child with the alleged meningitis is still there in the waiting room (next to the irritated man with atypical chest pain and the young woman with pelvic pains). He might well have a simple and reassuring history such as 24 hours mild fever, drinking fluids, not eating, lively at times, miserable but not clingy and perhaps some spots of some kind. On the history as given it could well be sorted out on the telephone, but to convince the parents that the exclusion of meningitis etc. is possible via British Telecom is a rare skill, though not impossible. No, the parents will be wanting the wisdom to emanate from the physical check, but to be convincing the GP might consider demonstrating the presence or absence of some physical signs. Accordingly:

'I have checked him over and there are no signs of meningitis.'

is not so effective as

'I can see he is miserable with the fever and catarrh, and you can see the back of his throat is a bit red. His ears look fine (sometimes that's where the infection lies) and the rash is the dry, scaly sort of eczema and a different problem. I know he's been sick a few times and not taken as much fluid as you'd like but he's not dehydrated because you can see his eyes are alert, the tongue moist and his skin is smooth and not dehydrated. All this suggests a simple viral infection....'

and might be expanded further if an explicit worry has been prised out:

'Meningitis makes them floppy rather than this nice tone and a pale bluish colour round the lips rather than this lovely pink. The meningitis rash is really purple not red, though it is not always there at all.'

Or, in the case of the atypical chest pain,

'Your heart sounds fine. I'm sure it's not that.'

is not as good as

'As I've said the pain you describe doesn't sound like heart trouble at all. Your blood pressure is normal, and listening to how the heart valves are going and checking your body to see how well it is pumping the blood are all normal. There is some tenderness around the ribs here – do you think that might be behind the pain? We might not be able to pinpoint the cause of this pain exactly, but we can still help ease it....'

If the plan fails

The patient is now feeling understood, having had a series of chances to put his or her worries across not just at the initial history-taking stage of the conversation but at several points thereafter. The patient has seen that the GP has come to a reasonable risk assessment because he or she can see the line of thinking the GP has taken and it is plausible. The GP has suggested what is much the most likely course of the situation, be it via natural recovery, some course of therapy, symptomatic relief or whatever. This too looks good to the patient but he or she notes, not being stupid, that the doctor is not prepared to guarantee the outcome. The GP merely expects it. And both the clinician and the patient need a sense of what to do if the doctor's expectations are not fulfilled.

The patient is being asked to

1. Identify the point where the prediction is failing

2. Know what to do.

Again, as with 'If you're worried, just get back in touch', the unconfident GP is liable to take the approach of 'I'd like to see you in a week/month/whatever to check you're all right'. This has many disadvantages even if it helps with the nervous medic's stress.

The first problem is the undermining of what has just been said, as the patient's train of thought might be 'If he's so sure it is not serious why does he want to see me again – why not do some more tests or send me to a specialist now?' thereby showing a considerable misunderstanding of the uncertainty issues we are considering.

The next is that the time frame could be wrong, as we have all seen patients who had a follow-up appointment for which they waited whilst obviously in trouble some time before. Or patients who were asked to return but did not, to their detriment, and did not understand the need to seek help.

And the use of time to see people who are mostly much better to pick up the few who are not is wasteful. This is the tendency of the inexperienced senior house officer (SHO) in an outpatient department, as well as the paternalistic GP.

Arguably some patients have to be given a shortish follow-up even whilst feeling well. Such a patient might have treatable, pre-symptomatic chronic disease and for whom things are going wrong, but they cannot of course know it without, say, a periodic blood test. But even here the GP should be able to put across to the patient his or her responsibility to have a blood test at a certain interval and in any case all primary care computer systems add the safety net of being programmed to disallow prescriptions to be filled (e.g. for warfarin) when checks are not done. Thus the GP absolutely minimises routine follow-up of self-limiting illness.

Fortunately we have just educated the patient about the problem he or she has and we have shared our knowledge, and the value we can place on it, with him or her. We therefore have a small jump to make to ask the patient to take responsibility for his or her own follow-up.

'The virus will probably get a bit worse before he gets better. He's likely to get more of a cough shortly. You'll have a couple of bad nights, I'm afraid. If his vomiting doesn't settle in a day or so, or if he has no wet nappies, or if the colour round his lips or face especially looks pale or ghastly get in touch – perhaps initially by phone.'

or

'The chest pain is likely to be a nuisance and I have to warn you we might not do brilliantly with it, but I am sure we can help. But since you came concerned about heart trouble and as you smoke and are a bit unfit let me know or contact the practice if the pain alters, or you get more short of breath especially on doing modest exercise.'

Yes, but can you trust the patient?

The patient likes you, you know. He or she wants to please you and wants to get better to make you feel good too. This motivation works alongside the patient's self-interest, and experience shows that a patient who leaves a consultation satisfied will try to follow the advice given. If the patient knows about his or her health problems and has a sense of empowerment, if the patient knows what to do about it and how to spot when the course of his or her health strays from the predicted path, then let the patient choose with confidence whether to involve you.

Conclusion

Reassurance is a difficult skill and we deal as clinicians with matters of such importance that other professions, who tend to influence us, have little to teach us. We need to deconstruct this section of the consultation into numerous parts and have a clear understanding of the problems at each stage; this saves time in the end. The GP develops skills to do this in depth, and examples of both suitable and unsuitable wording are included in this chapter. And it is all done with inner confidence and honesty!

References

1. Kaplan S, Greenfield S, Gandek B, *et al*. Characteristics of physicians with participatory decision making styles *Annals of Internal Medicine* 1996; **124**: 497–504.

2. Grol R, Whitfield M, De Maeseneer J, *et al*. Attitude to risk taking in medical decision making in British, Dutch and Belgian GPs *British Journal of General Practice* 1990; **40**: 134–6.

Further reading

Griffiths F, Green E, Tsouroufli M. The nature of medical evidence and its inherent uncertainty for the clinical consultation: qualitative study *British Medical Journal* 2005; **330**: 511–15. This is a study demonstrating how doctors are liable to create a myth of certainty whilst explaining their own uncertainty.

CHAPTER 9

Complaints and the imperfect GP

The pressure felt by GPs when they are the subject of a complaint can be disproportionate. It is difficult to rationalise so the consequence is that the fear of complaints distorts behaviour and decision making. We have a particular fear of the press, analysed here, and a tendency to drop into a defensive stance because of these factors. GPs are exhorted to know their boundary and to use their freedoms to define it. Finally, the virtues of team analysis of significant events are considered.

What might be the current, fashionable buzzwords around health care in the early years of this century? Certain words and phrases enter the enclosed world of health care from time to time, lasting a year or two and sometimes longer until a new insight appears. They arise mysteriously and are promoted with some vigour, generally by ministers anxious to be at the cutting edge of whichever reorganisation they preside over.

Past buzzwords might be 'team-working' and 'care in the community'. 'Patient pathways', 'stakeholders' and 'choice' have been more recent in-words. There are many others.

The early part of this century has sprouted the 'learning organisation', 'lifelong learning' (perhaps slightly passé, that one) and 'significant event analysis'. The last one is not really new either, but as the favoured son of 'critical incident analysis' the idea that the event does not have to be a big one, or have big consequences, to be worth analysing is quite fresh. These laudable words are an attempt to get us 'stakeholders' to view the task we face rather differently. We are to find ways of becoming more aware of our inadequacies and strive to overcome them. Naturally we are honour bound to work within our skill levels because this is the only safe approach for the patient and we must create systems to identify current learning issues for ourselves. We must find the way in which we learn best and use it, and make sure sufficient priority is given by the organisation for which we work to the job of learning (i.e. protected time). And we should be double-checking that when we have ticked the box and learnt something that we can show it has resulted in change – or at least produce the paperwork showing we made the effort. This would ideally create a spiral of increasing knowledge.

This is too tidy for many GPs. The picture seems to be of a virtuous doctor having a sort of colander of knowledge – 90 per cent solid, but to our regret it holds no water. We focus on the holes, but as soon as one set of holes is plugged someone shrieks that he or she has spotted a whole zone of inadequacies in another part of the colander. As the colander continues to leak, the received wisdom is that it is not possible to cover all the gaps and holes, and we should not expect to. But if the overall theory works – holds water, as it were – there should be a diminishing number of holes in our colander as time goes by. We become increasingly competent. So if all the clinicians followed these principles the total body of knowledge would be steadily increasing. It might be doing that, but at some cost to physician confidence.[1]

A system designed to demonstrate new gaps as soon as we sort one lot out is not inherently rewarding to the doctor. For each learning gap, whether it was a problem that affected a patient or one spotted at an earlier stage by a different method (of which there are very many), we must have a lot of happy patients whose needs we met from our existing knowledge and skill base. Sadly, these patients rarely reward us with some words of reassurance that might help us to cope – not praise for being an unusually good GP or a particularly nice person, but a thank you for an ordinary job well done would be pleasant. Instead we are trained to put ourselves in the dock for our imperfections, unaware of all those unsaid character references from patients. Perhaps I malign patients whose gratitude is in fact spoken but neither heard nor acknowledged by the doctor – we might not be good at accepting compliments.

But from a patient point of view we have moved on from the patrician to partner now. And this discomforting truth can be both a threat and a gain to medical confidence and decisiveness. The GP who is not sure what is expected of him or her finds it hard to identify and admit to his or her imperfections. The one who is more comfortable with being human is able to share with his or her partner, the patient, what is within the GP's power and what is not, without shame.[2] This chapter is about living with at least some of our defects.

The manner of the complaint

A long-term anxiety of GPs is the long list of agencies to which a complainant might turn. Complainants are expected initially to go to the practice, but if unsatisfied they have recourse to the Primary Care Organisation (PCO) and its mechanisms, and even beyond that the Health Services Ombudsman. The legal system might be involved, either the criminal justice or the civil courts, but when it is involved the NHS system stops. The General Medical Council (GMC), under heavy criticism in recent years, hears complaints that are sent to it, though its role is under close review. However, the statistical risk of being involved in a GMC complaint, or one that reaches open court, is very small for a GP and certainly less than one per working lifetime. Without minimising the alarm the prospect of these mechanisms being used against a GP causes, I will focus on the more everyday complaints practices handle and especially their impact on GP decision making. All the authorities like the defence societies report that well-handled complaints at practice level are most unlikely to progress, and over-defensive and unapologetic responses inflame the problem.[3] The method of communicating with complainants is much the same set of skills used in a consultation – listening, investigating, clarifying, explaining – with a low threshold for apologising. It is a myth that apologising implies accepting liability.[4]

I don't want to complain but I have a complaint

Any administrator who has run a complaints system is familiar with the patient or relative who wishes to make a complaint about a problem that has occurred, but dislikes the idea that what he or she wants to say is a formal 'Complaint'. It seems that patients believe that they can, by making the issue into a 'Complaint', trigger some kind of definitive reprimand to whoever was responsible, rather than just an investigation, and they do not always feel their issue is worth such drastic measures. Or perhaps they do want to see a consequence, but they do not want to make a big effort or are frightened of the consequences if they stir up trouble. These grumblers are sometimes inconsistent and lack confidence in seeing their gripe through logically; if a matter is minor then surely all they have to do is to say so.[5] If a matter is serious they should be honest about it and they have a duty, perhaps uncomfortably, to sort it. Consequently the administrator, perhaps in a practice the manager or the executive partner, has to decide if a complaint is 'serious'.

Anecdotally, doctors seem to accept the idea that every complaint is a complaint leading to a consequence of some kind. Why are we so insecure about them? Do we not have the same inconsistency of approach as patients?

It is curious how we feel we have to complain about ourselves in the absence of adverse patient comment. But in a way the very process of educational needs assessment seems like self-complaining. As discussed previously we are taught to do our own PUNs (patient's unmet needs) and DENs (doctor's educational needs) because the patients do not complain sufficiently and point out the faults that led to inadequate or sub-optimum care – areas that might have gone better. To draw a list of PUNs and DENs does not seem to take long – just look at last week's work. Surely no full week goes by in which nothing within one's power could have gone better? By doing the PUNS and DENS exercise we almost acknowledge that a patient should or could complain about something – as opposed to 'Complain' – probably at least weekly. But we should feel less bad about it; this does not reflect poor decision making. It reflects the impossible range of undifferentiated medicine. As it is most of us go through a whole professional lifetime without being sued, and many years between heavyweight 'Complaints'. Yet the shadow of these unlikely events in our working life darkens each day that we work. The final logic of this argument, if patients are our partners, is that we should encourage more feedback, including constructive criticism (complaints, not Complaints).

Insufficient patient complaints

The GP who declares that he or she must be doing all right because he or she gets very few complaints is a common, and comical, figure. Assuming this to be accurate and that the pompous doctor is truly not getting many complaints, none of the possible explanations reflects well on the clinician. What they are not is 'all right'. What they are not, a moment's thought would confirm, is acting in the patients' interest. They might be highly risk-averse and so tending to pass responsibility to colleagues all the time.

The latter point about not taking risks has a parallel in surgeons' league tables. The simple top-of-the-league surgeon, whose patients are most likely to survive the knife, might be operating on people who do not need it, and declining to operate on the ones in most trouble, who would benefit most but also carry the biggest risk. This is not the surgeon one necessarily wishes to consult, therefore. (So a more sophisticated analysis of risk is required to judge performance.[6]) Likewise it is quite possible that the GP with no complaints on file is not at all competent.

Patients rarely moan when a doctor passes them on from him or herself to another clinician, be it GP to consultant, specialist to specialist or GP to another healthcare professional. They know the attention to their problem is merited. But we know that sometimes the referrer could have coped a bit better, and not caused delay and used up limited resources by asking for a further opinion of some kind. The unconfident, risk-averse referrer is not acting in either the patient's or society's interest but the patient will not complain – they will sing the referrer's praises ('He knew exactly what to do – he sent me straight to Dr Smith'). However, they might be doing little or no work. This clinician is therefore not comparable to the average GP worried about his or her complaint volume. The GP might be so intimidating that his or her patients fear being open about any complaint. This is not just the Lancelot Spratts of the medical world.

The doctor (or nurse) exerts a considerable authority over the patient, especially the lower socio-economic groups, the less articulate and educated. It is easily forgotten when fearing the power of the patient who can complain or run to the press that the clinician might be viewed by the patient as holding even greater, terrifying, power. The clinician wishing to get helpful feedback, especially from disadvantaged groups, has to break down this barrier, which at first makes him or her absurdly vulnerable. It takes a lot of confidence.

Patients will remain reticent unless they are convinced their complaint does not affect their care. This is an even tougher barrier to get over, perhaps because a complaint does indeed affect their care; they are right. We all have experience of patients who have complained, and possibly without full justification in our eyes, and there is then an unresolved agenda between us. The fear of the patient is of retribution – worse care, perhaps not listening, not being available, or mean prescribing. In fact the observation is that the patient might be shepherded to another GP or colleague. Sometimes it is easier after a complaint to grant increased access to the more senior doctor whose experience allows the patient to be managed more happily without further complaints. Such eggshell-walking is surely unlikely to work in the patient's interest in the end, even if the senior GP is as a consequence more available. GPs might have no system to become aware of complaints or a manager who is as nervous as the patients about saying they have one.

Above all this is a management issue; but the partnership between manager and doctor is not always one of equals. If the personality of the GP is such that he or she feels responsible for any adverse event to one of his or her patient, even though they are just one of the team of advisers and workers, then this is a display of low confidence that is itself a DEN. Some doctors react with personal hurt and upset if they appeared to have played a part in an adverse event as if they are not part of a system, and so they over-react. If a GP is very sensitive, colleagues and timid office staff might be protective and reluctant to bring issues up (unless they are really too big to ignore) and so they are unlikely to devise systems that positively encourage complaints. The only person who can change this effectively is the lead doctor who has learned to delegate effectively.

So we know patients grumble informally, and we know we are imperfect because we try to identify our problems ourselves. Therefore, learning to accept mildly negative but constructive patient feedback by encouraging more of it, and gaining experience by using it regularly (so the doctor loses the fear of catastrophe), should strengthen us. Well-validated patient satisfaction surveys are a start.

The freedom of the press

The victim mentality that doctors and nurses display about complaints peaks with the possibility of the press getting hold of the story. But truly this does not stand up to rational argument and it is worth being a bit right-brained and logical about this, before one allows the possibility of adverse press coverage to deflate professional self-confidence.

Press coverage of medical issues is not wholly negative. There are many stories, loosely categorised as medical, that talk of new advances and services, breakthroughs, drugs and techniques, or give neutral advice, much more than tales of medical misdemeanours. The journalists' sources for these upbeat and feelgood stories are often the NHS press officers, the drug and healthcare industry and even the local trust board meetings, which tend to be relayed uncritically and so positively. One might ponder on the motivation behind press releases and the PR machine, and whether the front-line clinician is made more vulnerable to the increased expectations of the population. But that the press gives a lot of space to positive stories is measurably true.[7]

The negative press can arise from many sources.[8] It is an unusual Sunday that does not have some story about an aspect of the NHS that is reportedly struggling for lack of some resource – money, specialists, kit. Such tales will arise from an interest group, either professional or patient, feeding the newspaper with its side of the issue and it developing from there. 'Cancer service worst in Europe' might arise from a group of patients with a rare sort of cancer, or the clinicians looking after them, producing thin statistics showing how neglected they are by the vast and impersonal provider. This is preferably done by comparison with the private sector abroad, e.g. numbers of intensive therapy unit (ITU) beds, spending on new therapies, with the unspoken assumption that the comparator is better because it spends more and has more machines. Evidence to prove this is not always produced, a point the journalist might make in the latter paragraphs. This sort of story riles doctors but they should feel little inappropriate pressure because the story blows over. The main danger is the doctor feeling under siege from too many of these. But actually we cannot remember the sob story from last month, even though we were interested in it at the time, so surely the patient and the politician have even less chance of helpful recall.

The next type of negative coverage is a feature of an open society and the need for justice to be seen to be done. It is vital that the reporting of those rare but evil, dishonest or dangerous colleagues is encouraged, preferably at the trial stage but sometimes by journalistic exposure before the authorities know of the problem. This applies to all walks of life, and represents a public safety net. No doctor benefits from any attempt to curb this reporting; the public knows that Allitt is not representative of nurses, Shipman of GPs, or the Bristol team of heart surgeons. These few stories are huge and the acreage of paper granted to them accounts for much of the weight of negative stories.

It is the final type of negative coverage that hurts doctors and nurses. '"Doctor missed my cancer for months" – claims mother, 35' or 'Nurses too busy with paperwork to clean up Granny' giving the patient's view of a medical episode is the headline feared by the working GP or nurse. This type of story is not as common as we think, partly because the journalists have some sense that there is more to a story than this and in checking it out realise the truth is more mundane. The fear of libel is high and works to our advantage; the defence societies are adept at dousing stories.

Fame at last

All clinicians, certainly doctors, who have worked for very long have either missed a serious illness for a while or been part of a team that took more time than would be ideal to diagnose a serious illness. I had a young man with a painful shoulder that, it eventually emerged, was the presentation of a rare form of muscle cancer. There was little treatment for him once it was manifest. The family moved away to relatives.

When some time later a TV company rang one afternoon asking for an interview to 'give my side of the tragedy and defend myself against the charges of incompetence made by the parents' I had not heard from the family for a long time. Fortunately I took advice from the medical defence union, who advised that a) the TV producer was unlikely to let me actually broadcast anything helpful to my side, b) I could not speak to them anyway because I did not have the patient's permission, and so c) I must decline. The producer said the story was going out that day at 6 p.m. I declined to comment at all.

The story was never broadcast. The medical defence union pointed out that it was probably libellous and the company lawyers would have pulled the plug.

I had an anxious few hours. The system defended me. Tragically but unavoidably, the man died.

The individual GP has but a remote risk of being erroneously fingered by the irresponsible press. We have far more problems with poor reporting of science (witness the ignorance around MMR) than with unfounded accusations. And even when they appear, the reputation of the doctor named is rarely scratched for long.

So coldly, calmly, the confident GP should not fear the press. Fearing the press is like fearing being run over by a bus; yes it can happen, but it is so unlikely that all you have to do is avoid walking in front of one and you'll be fine. But, being human, the left brain is still nervous and upset, and one can but try to soothe it with logic rather than passion.

The consequence of the fear of complaints, aside from stress in the GP, is that we draw in our boundary, or practise defensively. Whilst there might be some virtues in this greater apparent clarity and care in delivery, it also shows how we struggle with our responsibilities.

119

It's not my job; I'm not covered (or paid) to do that

Most GPs cherish their independent status much as a dog does its place in front of the fire, and one of the attractions of the job is the belief that a doctor may set his or her own boundary. This is not just the physical boundary within which they accept patients; this is far more the boundary of the role. First, beyond the core work are both the defined (and paid for) enhanced services and the ill-defined (and unpaid) interests and skills of the GP, perhaps like acupuncture, counselling or other forms of care. However, there is a more interesting boundary within the core work. For instance, how far does a GP go in treating heart failure, obstetric problems, sexual health, bereavement, varicose veins or infant feeding problems? Some of these will have a boundary it would be difficult to argue over now – whilst 30 years ago you could still find GPs who did interventional obstetrics (i.e. forceps deliveries). This would now, for almost all of us, be inexcusable. Current management guidelines on the care of heart failure clearly prefer a specialist to start beta-blocker therapy but more and more GPs are gaining proficiency with these drugs – they remember the same consultant-only rule was once for ACE inhibitors after all. Bereavement therapy, where warranted, is frequently referred on though it is not a difficult counselling skill for the most part, and certainly we are all capable of it – if we are interested. And so on – the boundary of what we are doing in primary care is individually set by the GP, depending on his or her interest and skill rather than patient need necessarily. If there is a patient need and we do not wish or cannot provide it we can send them on elsewhere.

This perhaps contrasts with the secondary sector, which is clearer as to who does and should do what. The consultant, the manager or the commissioner sets the duties out in the end.

The problem in primary care is that these decisions about what to do, do not always result in the care being given elsewhere – whilst one GP might not feel able to do any simple bereavement counselling another might refer, but the third might not do either and the patient loses out.

It also becomes easy for us to say that writing a decent letter to the housing authority, routinely visiting dying patients, liaising with a school, or double-checking a drug addict's sick note are not part of our job. The fear of getting involved in the daily psycho-social mayhem we witness might be from time constraints, or fear of getting blamed, or a stereotyped weary frustration with patients.

But more worrying is the inflexible application of a PCO's or consultant's views on what we should and should not do. A chest physician might say all patients with chronic obstructive pulmonary disease (COPD) in the severe category should be seen in their clinic, but a GP might well be competent to manage them. If so it is surely defensible to do so. GPs competent to do this but uncertain of their boundary might feel such a statement is an absolute, they have no choice and the fact that the patient waits three months (and is then nurse managed) is not their problem – they are doing as the system tells them.

Declaring oneself (wrongly) as 'not covered to do that' can be a judgement on the other members of the team. The implication is that the team will criticise the hapless GP who steps beyond the undrawn line. There is a fear that 'something might go wrong', although many such jobsworths find it hard to describe what, exactly, might go wrong, and why if it does the blame will be focused on them. This indictment of senior clinicians and managers has to be spotted and handled well, because it eats away at us lower orders. The team that has a culture of 'you're not covered to do that' is nurturing nervous doctors. The team which recognises that individual clinicians need a clear idea of their competences more than their job description, that they then act within them and in the patients' interests, and use good communication and safety netting techniques, will grow confident and strong.

The Ministry of Defensive Medicine

Taking major professional responsibility is one of the features, and prides, of independent GPs, working as they are within their boundaries and with their patients. Much of the scariest responsibility we take is in pronouncing that someone is fit and well. This simple joyful message to the patient, who might not understand the profound skill and responsibility that underlies it, carries a risk. The risk is not large, because we are all well trained and know our stuff, but there is something peculiarly unforgivable about missing something sinister and giving erroneous reassurance. We are allowed to subject our patients to anxiety, radiation, expense, drugs, pain and indignity in the cause of not missing things. Yet, in so far as the effort produces nothing we did not know, we need not have done the tests and so get the decision to investigate wrong a lot of the time. There seems no need to apologise, because the absence of bad news at the end of it all is so overwhelming for the patient that he or she forgives us everything (and anyway we are so nice and plausible about it). This applies, as Balint noted in 1952, to physical illnesses but not psychological ones. The doctor who overlooks a barn door-sized depression is not seen as negligent just because he or she focused for several months on the anaemia caused by self-neglect from the untreated mental illness. Indeed, even if the patient is spotted as being depressed this might still not be considered adequate explanation for the accompanying anaemia, and the endoscopies are lined up. The double standard continues now, with the practice of defensive medicine being more the problem of the physicians and surgeons than the psychiatrists.

We all seem to practise defensive paperwork nowadays, the volume of modern medical records (paper or computerised) being testament to that.

This is another boundary issue. The decision-making GP who sees the patient is aware of the level of support he or she might get from peers in the event of problems, and might perceive this to be inadequate. The chain of command in clinical care is not an efficient military one, where responsibility is ultimately taken quite high up. (The lower orders in the military's valley of death are, as we know, not there to reason why, theirs is just to do or die....[9])

In health care the lower orders – you and I – are professional and capable of a surprising amount of autonomy and responsibility. We do reason why. But if the boundary at the edge of our capability is patrolled by an unsupportive hierarchy we will tend to draw it in, and patients get passed beyond it into the zone marked *Other People's Problems* or possibly *Protocol-Driven Care* – somewhere safe, where our judgement is not really needed. The Secretary of State himself can be relied upon to make warm and soothing noises about the clinical professions in general, but he is unlikely to stand up and defend an individual within it for doing his or her job. This culture trickles down and the poor bloody NHS infantry are left feeling alone. Given the shame that is perceived to tip down on the doctor who missed a physical problem, it is not surprising that doctors reach for the body armour of defensive medicine. If it was any good at deflecting flak, it might be justified.

That the pursuit of error-free medicine, by covering all angles and remembering all possibilities, is wasteful is self-evident. But the stuff breeds on itself. How many patients have had a collection of investigations for some symptom or sign that throws up a completely different problem, such as an abnormal parameter on the blood tests, which the GP had not asked for and did not want to know? The decision then to delve further into the laboratory abnormality is inevitable because neither patient nor GP can relax with this new knowledge alone. We have to know more 'just in case', although we are rarely sure just in case what, exactly. No protocol seems to help; the patient does not fit into a category and is not yet ready to fit into a box. But our fear drives the process on and it takes some confidence and experience to call a halt to it. There is morbidity and even mortality attached to this process, as well as the consumption of resources better used elsewhere and massive patient anxiety – a kind of overkill. It arises because of a misunderstanding of the Wilson screening criteria which point out (amongst other things) that we should only look for illness in a pre-symptomatic stage that is treatable and whose natural course is understood.[10] A good example of this process of overkill is cervical cytology systems, especially when they are done too often (recent NICE report),[11] and the tendency to worry about cholesterol levels in young hypertensive patients despite a complete lack of proven benefit in treating them even when levels are high – but it remains on the guidelines for hypertension care.[12,13] So we do it and keep measuring it and doing it in different ways and advising on low-fat diets.

We are all subject to defensive protocols and even the strong GP might not be able to question that, and perhaps will only try if insufficient resource prevents their use. But if the clinical situation is analysed carefully the option to continue with uncertainty is still important to consider and share. Skilfully done, the GP can practise this safely and yet sleep at night.

Moving on from mistakes

It used to be advised to doctors that they must ensure that all their mistakes were big ones, and that they all get properly buried. Yet so far in this chapter we have discussed digging up our mistakes and looking at them in a counter-intuitive attempt to bolster confidence in our performance. The culture shift moves on to an analysis of what is happening in the patient's care, what might have gone better and perhaps what might one, as an individual, like to change. This to the unconfident sounds like a confessional, like an Alcoholics Anonymous (AA) meeting of reformed clinicians.

So long as the no-blame rule is agreed and followed, the process of rooting through the sequence of events that led to a calamity can be empowering. The team involved is, first of all, defined even if they had not perceived themselves to be a team. They are obliged by the exercise to empathise with the patient, always a good thing. The experience of having a good leader for the discussion and analysis is that the people involved have a clearer knowledge of their role and that of the others, and can safely chip in with ideas and thoughts to make changes. If the ground rules for significant analysis are followed (see box) it just becomes part of professional life.[14]

Some rules for a significant event analysis discussion

- The object is to learn and never to blame.

- The event need not be big: a missed appointment or a broken ECG machine might be the basis for a team discussion on exactly the process needed to ensure smooth appointments or getting the ECG machine repaired (or not breaking it in the first place) – with immediate patient benefit. But clearly an unexpected death or predictable drug abreaction needs analysis too. Some 'difficult' situations, like an abusive drunk in a waiting area, might at first seem worth logging as an event but the discussion might not generate workable solutions; careful consideration of the topic is needed.

- There is value in looking at an example of what went well, a positive event, whose lessons could be carried to other parts of the system.

- Confidentiality needs to be tight.

- Minutes, however, need to be kept and agreed.

- Action points might feed into Personal Development Plans (PDPs).

- All team members should be encouraged to speak and be listened to, and all team members should help identify significant events.

- Going for a sociable drink afterwards is acceptable.

The conclusion the team arrives at must be to look for their mistakes systematically and only expect their care to be 95–99 per cent acceptable. Any more and they are deluded, and any less and they are either over-critical or they (and their patients) have a problem whose root needs finding.

They must grasp their mistakes as opportunities and devise ways of safely sharing them, rather than use them for self-flagellation. The average patient is a forgiving person and if the concepts of partnership are believed then the team will make progress without fearing error.

They should read newspapers and not really believe them, just like everyone else, and take advice when they are approached by the media (generally to keep quiet).

The dangers of defensive medicine are clear and need understanding even if one cannot stop its practice entirely.

And the doctor is aware of the level of support the hierarchy can give, which is limited, but he or she understands and is comfortable about it.

Conclusions

Many of us receive insufficient complaints so the unfamiliarity scares us. The system teaches us to fear them but this discussion suggests we can use them for planning, learning and changing so long as we know that we are not isolated. We must be confident in saying so when the complainant has no case. We also fear the press, but this too needs more rationalisation because we want our patients to be realistic about us GPs rather than expect miracles. Health issues will always sell papers and the ownership of those issues is with all of us, not just the professions.

References

1. Jain A, Ogden J. General practitioners' experiences of patients' complaints: a qualitative study *British Medical Journal* 1999; **318**: 1596–8.

2. Cheraghi-Sohi S, Bower P, Mead N, *et al*. What are the key attributes of primary care for patients? Building a conceptual 'map' of patient preferences *Health Expectations* 2006; **9(3)**: 275–84.

3. Baker R. Learning from complaints about general practitioners *British Medical Journal* 1999; **318**: 1567–8.

4. Lamb R. Open disclosure: the only approach to medical error *Quality and Safety in Health Care* 2004; **13**: 3–5.

5. Schlesinger M, Mitchell S, Elbel B. Voices unheard: barriers to expressing dissatisfaction to health plans *The Milbank Quarterly* 2002; **80**: 709–55.

6. Sutton R, Bann S, Brooks M, *et al*. The Surgical Risk Scale as an improved tool for risk-adjusted analysis *British Journal of Surgery* 2002; **89**: 763–8.

7. Karpf A. *Doctoring the Media* London: Routledge, 1988.

8. Ali NY, Lo TY, Auvache VL, *et al*. Bad press for doctors *British Medical Journal* 2001; **323**: 782–3.

9. Tennyson A. 'The Charge of the Light Brigade', 1854.

10. Wilson JMG, Jungner G. *Principles and Practice of Screening for Disease* Geneva: World Health Organization, 1968.

11. Sasieni P, Adams J, Cuzick J. Benefits of cervical screening at different ages: evidence from the UK audit of screening histories *British Journal of Cancer* 2003; **89(1)**: 88–93.

12. Williams B, Poulter NR, Brown MJ, *et al*. The BHS Guidelines Working Party guidelines for management of hypertension: report of the Fourth Working Party of the

British Hypertension Society, 2004 – BHS IV *Journal of Human Hypertension* 2004; **18**: 139–85.

13. Sever PS, Dahlöf B, Poulter NR, *et al*. ASCOT investigators. Prevention of coronary and stroke events with atorvastatin in hypertensive patients who have average or lower-than-average cholesterol concentrations, in the Anglo-Scandinavian Cardiac Outcomes Trial – Lipid Lowering Arm (ASCOT-LLA): a multicentre randomised controlled trial *Lancet* 2003; **361**: 1149–58.

14. Pringle M, Bradley CP. Significant event auditing: a user's guide *Audit Trends* 1994; **2**: 701–13.

CHAPTER 10

Personal organisation and effectiveness

This chapter starts to look at the basic issues of how GPs, sometimes decisive and clear minded in the consultation, find that organising themselves is a problem. During the day they are buffeted by demands to complete paperwork and attend to tasks that do not have an immediate relevance to the patient in front of them. We discuss what a manager is, and what happens when you cannot find the tendon hammer. We look at the perils of prioritising and the need to minimise the tendency of decisions to linger. We touch on delegating skills and compare the skills needed in delegating to staff and patients alike.

How do you manage?

The abuse directed at hapless managers, either in particular or in general, is shocking. Every political opposition finds a disingenuous way of counting 'managers' (such as taking total NHS employees and deducting the number of doctors and nurses, thus including all staff who are not actually on wards, including catering, secretarial, laboratory, maintenance and payroll) – and decrying the resulting number as an appalling waste of taxpayers' money on 'pen pushers'. The cheap headline implies that the presence of a manager in the system is evidence of some kind of inefficiency, and should be stamped out. An outbreak of management is spotted – and pressure put on to sort it out before any harm is done, like finding legionnaires' disease in the water system.

Even primary care clinicians are wont to collude in this, to their shame and detriment, never mind the patients.

Doctors' cultural differences with managers are well documented but it starts very often with them not actually knowing what a manager is. Even GPs with their close working relationship with managers, whom they are probably actually paying themselves, seem to get muddled about what the role is. The confusion in their minds is often between managers and administrators. An administrator is the person who ensures the surgery rooms are cleaned, stocked and usable, possibly by delegating to cleaners, receptionists and nursing staff the details and ensuring consumables like paper sheets are available. They are the people who operate the system created by managers. The manager, from the point of view of this chapter, is the person who has planned the clinic timetable and monitors the systems for appointments, staffing and communications. In a small primary care team the 'manager' might well do the administration stuff him or herself, but a larger practice will often separate the roles more distinctly.

When a problem occurs the doctor might well wish to sound off to a manager, but the more junior administrator might have been the problem. Or the culprit might be another team member, like the GP him or herself.

Whatever happens to medical equipment?

A minor inefficiency of any clinical setting is the disappearance of everyday desktop equipment, like the tendon hammer, the pad of sick notes or the ophthalmoscope with the decent batteries. The reaction of the doctor, from observation, is usually an irritated demand to the receptionist to find the original or a replacement, and he or she might well approach the manager who will not have a clue and has better things to do.

The doctor meanwhile 'borrows' from another room what is needed or what will do as a substitute, thereby deferring rather than solving the problem.

The receptionist after 20 minutes buzzes through and says they cannot find the item.

The doctor says that's alright.

The administrator might be aspiring to higher levels of running the organisation, to management proper as it were. As with the McDonald's restaurant managers, whose training invariably starts with a number of tiresome shifts sizzling burgers and pumping milkshakes, the NHS manager – in primary or secondary care – will know how toilet rolls are ordered but pretty soon, he or she hopes, will rise above being the one actually phoning the supplier.

Tellingly, until about the mid-1970s hospitals were run by administrators rather than managers, and the implication was that the function of the small-office staff was merely to service the needs of patients and their clinicians (doctors, really). The direction of the organisation and its central purpose was set by the senior doctors. Bringing in a management culture, strengthened by the reforms of the 1990s especially, appears to have brought stronger concepts of corporate identity and accountability.

Likewise the size of the management agenda in a practice has increased hugely in the last 20 years, with all GPs employing managers now and bigger practices having a team of office staff; in the early 1980s this would have seemed very top heavy. These staff are necessary to carry through the more complex agenda and administer the more complex systems any practice has, like data processing, clinical and corporate governance methods, training, health and safety, employment, strategic planning and financial control. All these management activities are much more sophisticated than 20 years ago. And as with the rest of the NHS, managers have been transferred in from the private (or other, such as the military) sectors, and of course bring useful skills. What all managers, and especially these transferees, find hard is establishing their relationship with the doctors.

Two hats and putting patients first

There is a conflict of interest in the waiting room.[1] On the one hand the kindly doctor-doctor wants the patients who, regrettably but inevitably have to use the waiting areas, to find the experience comfortable and friendly. He or she wants to provide well-lit, pleasant surroundings, informative notice boards, comfortable, maintained seating and clean loos. On the other hand the business-doctor, keen to maximise profits, does not wish to invest more in the room than he or she has to because there is no return. A business-doctor knows that spending at the minimum required to satisfy the regulatory authorities is the most cost-effective level. Further investment (a smarter environment) is not rewarded by increased business and hence profits, because patients register with doctors due to other factors than waiting room comfort such as locality, family, inertia, gender and so on. The most cynical doctor might even consider that too much comfort in the area will attract too much work (existing patients will want to come to him or her more) without an increase in income (since he or she is not paid per patient attendance).

127

This becomes a rather personal management issue. The doctor as employer might have chosen to set the budget for overheads (the costs a practice incurs just for existing, even if it has no activity). The overall budget for overheads would include the waiting area facilities and everything else (like staff, energy costs, and so on). Such a practice has a manager. If, however, they meet to instruct their manager to buy new chairs from a particular brochure, they are employing an administrator.

It is only human for the profit-taking doctor to expect involvement in the management when decisions might be made that ultimately impact on whether the doctor's holiday this year is spent in a Mediterranean hotel or under canvas in Yorkshire. The personal management issue for the doctor is in deciding how much involvement and effort the manager and/or executive partner has, and how much the doctor can trust him or her to work in the practice's financial interest.

The professionalism of doctors comes from their willingness at least sometimes to act in the patients' interest but against their own, in the sense that they might do things that bring no thanks or financial reward but which help patients. Is it unethical to have a drab and unfriendly waiting room? Having a comfortable surgery is one example of this simple dilemma; visiting after evening surgery out of kindness rather then necessity might be another. A third might be processing tiresome paperwork efficiently.

Decisiveness in management terms for an effective GP can often mean delegating and trusting to others. However, there is always a proportion of GP work that is not face-to-face patient contact, and yet is unavoidable.

Being efficient on paper

The problem of priorities

There is a time management myth that the way to sort out your day and be most efficient is to prioritise tasks. This idea suggests that you can work out what is most important, make sure that that is done first and go steadily down the list so at the end of the day the crucial work is definitely done, plus some of the less vital tasks, but no time has been lost on trivia.

This advice suffers from sounding glib, but we might try to prioritise a GP's day, as shown on Table 10.1.

Table 10.1: Prioritising a GP's day

Category A	■ Seeing all those patients booked in, or as emergencies ■ Necessary visits ■ Partners' meeting ■ Clinical correspondence, results, phone calls
Category B	■ Audits, Quality and Outcomes Framework (QOF) data collection ■ Teaching activities ■ Preparation for appraisals, own professional education work
Category C	■ Coffee break ■ Non-clinical patient-related paperwork (housing, insurance, requests for information from government departments and so on) ■ Other meetings (e.g. Practice-Based Commissioning, chat with pharmacy adviser)
Category D	■ Tidying room or computer ■ Surveys and Primary Care Organisation (PCO) paperwork ■ Personal things like popping to the bank, ringing the hairdresser ■ Look at Practice Development Plan (PDP)

Note: the point of this is not to suggest these as sensible priorities of the modern GP. We might all set different ranking orders.

This does not work, however, because of the:

■ continual effort in prioritising

■ sense that some jobs are worth doing 'only if there's time'.

We need to accept that an item of work is actually either worth doing or not.

The first difficulty of a priority list is in the inter-relation of the tasks. For example, whilst tidying is a low priority if we fail to do it, if we later cannot find the letter from the cardiologist we seek this then becomes a highly urgent and disruptive task when a patient comes to discuss it. If we do not make time to look at the Development Plan the next partners' meeting is ineffective. Items move around the list and we keep having to adjust it.

The further problem is that some items are really deserving of a priority so low we should not do them at all, but we do not identify them as such and just do them badly: surveys, some phone calls, some correspondence. We have been indecisive about our use of time. This might be a failure of delegation or a failure to decide clearly if something is worthwhile and so we procrastinate. We create yet another category, E!

The logic of this is that there should be only two categories of task: worth doing and not worth doing. If it is not, then clearly one should not do it. If it is, then either one does it or ensures that someone else does it. If there is a category of work in between, then there is a constant sense of incompletely finishing, of guilty work that might be useful yet is left undone.

Do it now, and face the fearful

The time management expert's clichés of 'only pick a piece of paper up once' and 'tackle the job you are resisting most by picking it up first' might have wisdom but in a normal GP's life they do not seem to be panaceas either. This type of advice can sound like 'be strong and pull your socks up; no one else will do it for you'.

The GP struggling with his or her workload is usually referring to that work which is other than face-to-face contact: within limits the sense of pressure from uncompleted task lists of unloved 'paperwork' rather than abandoned patients lingering in an unfinished clinic. Much of this part of our work is not amenable to being shifted smoothly from the in-tray to the out-tray in a neat, scheduled time slot. A result of uncertain importance might await the patient returning a call, a clinical problem one wishes to discuss awaits the team meeting or a chance to speak to a consultant colleague (three attempts so far), and a legal report awaits proper evidence of consent before being despatched. Stuff lingers and, though we can minimise it, there is always some of this. Yet GPs do seem to vary in the quantity of 'pending' they hold and this does suggest that there is room for improvement.

Nevertheless there are some tasks that are best done almost as soon as they are generated because then they are done in less time. A referral letter done freshly at or just after a consultation will need less time as one will not need to refresh oneself of the case.

Minutes written just after a meeting likewise will take a short time only.

The task that many doctors seem to allow to linger is the unresolved clinical problem. The sense that they should look something up, check in the patient's distant past record, or have a serious think about the issues in the case is of course an attempt to minimise the uncertainty we live with. This case needs a brief, focused burst of energy to move it on. If this is severely time limited ('I will spend ten minutes checking out if that headache is really migrainous') the deadline will ensure, for confident GPs, that they achieve to the limit of their capacity.

The value of a signature

Jokes about bad handwriting aside, the signature of a doctor or nurse is required on a very considerable amount of documentation.

20,000 offences taken into consideration

As a young GP I was reported to the Health Authority or whatever structure it was called at that moment in the late 1980s by a pharmacist. My signature had been felt to be too easily forged, having degenerated sadly over the preceding months. It was never legible, consisting of a curly open loop and a complex undulating line, with a half return to the left, pretending to underline it and so round it off. But the squiggle had fallen off and barely the loop remained, like an upturned 'Q' with a faint tailing off indicating that there were more letters that should be there, but are for the moment kept secret.

Pleading guilty, a back-of-the envelope calculation of the work I'd done since qualifying suggested that perhaps they should pass sentence knowing that there were perhaps 20,000 other offences to be taken into consideration.

I was gently reprimanded rather than formally punished and my signature to this day is a little more complex....

The problem of the shoddy signature arises because one delegates to others the task of producing much paperwork (in GPs' case repeat prescriptions) and trusts them, and in effect the signature is an act of trust in them too. As the volume of the paperwork is great, the speed at which the signature is written rises proportionately. But of course the doctor's responsibility is to sign only those pieces of paper that warrant it, and that means checking.

Yet all GPs find themselves being asked to sign pieces of paper authorising things, like ambulance journeys, certain investigations, certain prescriptions, letters, sick notes and the like – which on occasion they know little about. Either they have not understood the piece of paper when it is presented because the thing is new to them, or they normally understand it but on occasion they are doing it for a patient they don't know or a colleague who is not available for the moment. The clerical staff just request a signature, and the harassed, and for the moment singularly unconfident, doctor weighs up the time spent sorting it out against the opportunity cost (i.e. what he or she would have done whilst looking into the need for the signature, like deal with the next patient). These are dangerous moments when they involve drugs and tests, and potentially wasteful in all cases.

The desire to minimise inconvenience to the hovering staff member and the distant patient is strong, and so is the desire to appear in control. Nevertheless to outsiders it appears odd how GPs will usually sign something under pressure.

Such demands for the clinicians' signature can be seen as a complex management problem that might arise from a past error or might simply be mysterious. Not infrequently procedures demanding ponderous paperwork have arisen from past problems and might even be legislated into working practice (like controlled drugs). On other occasions there might be a bureaucratic problem that needs cracking, and the hurried doctor needs to recognise that here the manager can help. The GP who is genuinely in control can identify the really valuable paperwork from the rest because he or she has understood the history of the system. Unconfident GPs get cross with it, and might haughtily ignore forms and such, to their own and their patients' detriment.

Delegation and asking other people to do things

We see the clearest split of all between the decisive and the indecisive in this everyday interaction. Doctors who know their own role and the group goals will also be good at this and will do it in an entirely forgettable way; episodes of good delegation and effective working with others happen all the time and go by without being remarked upon. But we all remember the times when we were dumped on, the time when a request felt wrong or rude or unreasonable. Especially if we felt we had to comply with the request and sort out the issue in question. This might be a grievance that dominates us, like a patient complaint, irrational but emotive.

Language is crucial in the task of getting others to do things, from the way a team member or fellow doctor is addressed (first names? jokily?) to the courtesy of the actual words we use. There has to be knowledge of the other party's job and capabilities but also his or her schedule, resources and back-up. For instance, GPs (and even more so hospital doctors) are notorious for sending weepy patients with housing issues to social workers, but social workers are not counsellors or housing officers, even if they know a man who is.

Everyone's worried

At a joint educational event between clinicians and social work trainees some years ago there was a case presented of a single mum, who had several children, who smoked 40 fags a day and couldn't sleep. The clinicians, doctors, were appalled by the smoking and honed in on this as the main issue for her and the children. The body of social workers took the 40-a-day habit as a sign of appalling stress requiring stress-management techniques and were, to the clinicians, too forgiving of the smoking habit. I don't recall anyone solving the sleep issue.

A common misunderstanding of cultures between doctors and some of the other caring professions is of urgency or timing. The junior doctor knows (or ought to know) that if asked to come to the ward now then the request means come now, not in an hour. Urgency to the social worker might well mean taking the case to the next allocation meeting next week. Primary care has a different timescale from our secondary colleagues; urgency means same day perhaps or even the same hour to a GP but, unless it is a crashing emergency, urgency to an outpatient department will necessarily mean when the specialist next has a clinic. This is a construct of the system and not really amenable to change but is amenable to understanding.

The GP might have the mobile phone number of his or her hospital colleague but also knows when it is reasonable to use it. Secretaries can be a good source of intelligence for finding out when it is convenient to talk to such colleagues and can also sometimes answer the question you were going to ask their boss. In practice all GPs find the exercise of discussing urgency with specialists gives mixed results – some say it is urgent if the GP says it is urgent, while others can more confidently make up their own mind. And some of course do not hear our anxiety at all.

Delegating to whom, exactly?

The real difficulties for doctors appear to be the question of where the responsibility lies. The art (and it is not a science) of delegation is one of the most difficult and scary things we do. The theory is easy. You can delegate as a GP or doctor those tasks that are suitable by having a subordinate who is sufficiently trained and supported to do it. But if it goes wrong you carry the can. And if you keep checking, because of this knowledge that you are ultimately responsible, you will create masses of work for yourself, and the person to whom you are delegating will be uncomfortable with the sense of lack of trust. On the other hand if you don't support the person in his or her task at all, because you want him or her to feel trusted and competent, he or she will be unhappy as well. It is really difficult to get this right. It might be helpful to think about this by looking at tasks delegated to various categories of colleagues.

Delegating to the secretary

Numerous capabilities of office staff are underused. GPs find themselves: preparing reports (with questions like 'When did you last see the patient?'); collecting data for audits; making individual decisions about non-attenders rather than policies; phoning for and chasing results; looking for articles, information or facts; preparing rotas, timetables and schedules; and more.

Little of this was on the university curriculum in their professional training.

You might feel the secretary could or should be able to write certain kinds of letter without them being dictated or written by the GP first. The key will be to ask if he or she feels able to do it, and to listen very carefully to the answer. What the GP wants to do will be to delegate the matter and forget it, moving on to the next job, but a less than confident response from the secretary must be spotted or it will go wrong. This does not mean the job should not be passed on but impediments need identifying and considering, be they time, training, resources or dyslexia. Some are solvable issues and some are not. The issue might well be confidence alone and the task of the doctor who still hopes to escape the chore of these letters will be to discuss the level of supervision the secretary is comfortable with, which means open discussion and involving the manager and other GPs in the group. The timescales need agreeing and then the work can commence. Everyone knows where they stand.

A decision to pass some work on to the secretary needs to be realistic, showing an understanding of the demands on his or her time, priorities and timescales.

Skilful delegation of work to office staff is central to the confident GP's perform-ance and self-preservation. It takes more than being nice at Christmas to have a good working relationship though.

Delegating to the nurse, the healthcare assistant and other clinical staff

Delegation is allowing the colleague to do something without close supervision, i.e. discussion of each case as it goes on. The work is possibly subject to audit but not every aspect every time.

We reach the same problem with office staff in finding that the doctor might well have many duties that are suitable for delegation, except that there is a multitude of confounding factors.

The GP who could hand work over is all too conscious of the line of responsibil-ity still. He or she can see a line of advantages to offloading: his or her time is better spent; the junior needs education and experience; the work is dull.

But holding back is something even confident GPs do for a variety of reasons. One is obviously they might not have a junior colleague yet up to the task, or the assessment of that might be incomplete or someone else's responsibility, so it is not yet clear what can be passed on. Another is that patients appreciate continuity of care and in the exercise of a minor task within the capability of the other staff the patient is more content with the (senior) GP he or she knows. This gives positive feedback to us and we all welcome the spiritual nourishment. Smart doctors recognise that if they fill their week with high-intensity, difficult medicine, which takes them to their intellectual and skill limit all the time, they will swiftly collapse from exhaustion. Regular encounters with the mundane in medicine are important for the sanity of most experienced and confident GPs; indeed, they keep them so.

All this aside, we do sometimes need to trust our colleagues, whether nurse, regis-trar or therapist, and having identified something you want them to do the clini-cian–clinician discussion will need to involve many of the same elements shown in good patient–clinician communication. There will be a listening phase before the proposal, an assessment of confidence as much as skill, and a discussion of follow-up intensity and method. There is a safety net to be agreed with the other party. Open questions ('How do you feel things are going?') will work better before closed ones ('Do you think you should be doing x now?'), which carry assumptions about what the colleague ought to be capable of and that might make him or her nervous or, worse, cavalier. Junior clinicians' development will depend on this sort of conversation going well, and if they learn to talk honestly then they will have achieved much, even if they are not quite ready for doing something new.

Once the agreement to delegate is made, it means releasing them from close supervision and initially both parties will be anxious. Wise GPs feels the agree-ment is based on sound evidence and understanding, and bottle up their anxiety by whatever means they can. It is a tough role.

But checking behaviour by GPs of their colleagues and juniors is an extremely undermining strategy, and damages their budding confidence. We all see it: the doctor who can't relax unless he or she has double-checked work done by colleagues. This might be inspecting a dressing, cross-checking a protocol to ensure it has been fully followed without short cuts, or reading the colleague's records some time after his or her consultation with the GP's patient. This can even be seeing the patient again, unscheduled, just to reassure him or herself that all is as it should be. Nervous checking behaviour is easily rationalised internally by the knowledge that it is in the patient's interest, and that they are carrying the can anyway. That the colleague finds it unsettling, at least, or undermining and sapping, at worst, is viewed as something the colleague should get over, as if the 'delegatee' is being unprofessional in some way in resenting the assumption that his or her work always needs checking. It takes some judgement to avoid doing this but there are sound reasons why doctors have to allow some autonomy to their protégées. That they will one day be senior is obvious. But just as secretaries who know that all spelling errors will be sorted by their boss won't bother to spell-check, so the clinical workers who know they are always going to be checked will, being human, not feel they have to take quite the responsibility they should. *The compulsive checking GP will do his or her patients no favours by burning out at a young age and do his or her future patients no good by not allowing colleagues and the training grades to flourish.* There is a balance between tolerating small errors of no lasting consequence by not checking everything, and undermining junior colleagues by expecting them to do everything the senior does and seeing them fail. If errors of lasting consequence occur, of course it was a misjudgement to delegate, and the senior clinician has some responsibility there – which is why he or she is paid more. Finally, it is humbling to realise that one learns from the junior clinician, who might actually be better at certain matters, or has a different but equally valid way of doing things. Insisting on everything being as one wishes is not team playing.

Delegating to the patient

If there is a simple theme to this volume it is the value of working with patients and not only asking them to take on some responsibility for the shared decisions and care of their health but also nurturing an atmosphere in which this is expected. The capability of the patient is easily underestimated. Related more to the patient's personality than educational attainment, the ease with which patients accept a level of responsibility will of course vary. But the successful GP will assume he or she can handle some responsibility at least and allow the reins of control to go a bit slack; patients are asking us to do a bit less problem solving and we should seize the chance to pass our anxieties back to them. Therefore delegating an aspect of care beyond one's own practice or team should trigger the idea that the patient could take this on him or herself. The line of responsibility, the Boundary, needs to be understood here.

Conclusions

Denigrating managers is to misunderstand them. They are no more incompetent than the doctors, and that means the whole range of competence is seen. The pragmatic view is to work to understand them and therefore with them. This applies to the ones the doctors employ and the ones in the PCOs.

Budgets are not simple blocks of money and visualising them in that way is unhelpful. We pay managers to do that bit. But the level to which we delegate to managers will vary – what the manager would ask for is consistency.

Time management solutions for GPs can be simplistic. Efficient and decisive GPs will be able to decide whether a task is important before considering when or how; if the task then is important then they need skills to delegate where possible. This is akin to consultation skills, which is fortunate because the patient might be in the team dealing with the issue.

References

1. Peacock S, Ruta D, Mitton C, *et al.* Using economics to set pragmatic and ethical priorities *British Medical Journal* 2006; **332**: 482–5.

Further reading

Forster M. *Get Everything Done* London: Hodder & Stoughton, 2000.

Swanwick T (ed.). *The Management Handbook for Primary Care* London: RCGP, 2004.

CHAPTER 11

Coping with colleagues

I don't suffer from stress. But I think I might be a carrier.

This chapter builds on the previous one to help uncertain and indecisive GPs be more effective in the various teams in which they work. A fairly deep understanding of the dynamics in a team is essential. Many problems of team-working are discussed here, with the intention that readers will consider which appear to apply to them and therefore what changes would be useful.

The second part of this chapter acknowledges the need for rationed health care and touches on the GP's duty to support this.

Finally we discuss a little about the introduction of new ideas and the communication techniques needed.

I'd like to see the doctor, please

Your appointment system does not work. This is true, I know, because no known system is perfect or anywhere near it, and should it not be true then please share this with everyone else and collect your Nobel Peace Prize. Perhaps by way of illustration we can discuss the problems of appointment systems and the ways they can be improved.

Some of the frustrations of sorting out complicated modern management issues mirror the consultation. Yet the recent changes in our relationship with patients in the privacy of our consulting room have been criticised because they make us too managerial.[1] However, we need to be pragmatic, not least in an era of performance-related pay.

I don't like Mondays

Why is it that all front-line clinicians find more emergencies occur on Mondays than any other day? Logic suggests that feverish children, suicidal teenagers and wheezy pensioners should be evenly distributed through the week, but primary and secondary care consistently experience a Monday peak.

We accept a seasonal and diurnal variation in health; these are facts of planetary geography. But the length of a week is not determined by geography or genetics, though some might say it is divinely directed. Much of the rural developing world doesn't recognise one day as different from another in fact. It seems unlikely that they experience greater ill health every seventh day.

This is organisational, cultural, psychological. We discuss the need for asking for help over the weekend when we have reflective time. We've visited Granny, we've discussed the depression, we've panicked with the child and we've recovered from the hangover. Our patience runs out on Monday. The same problem is experienced by plumbers and the man who fixes the roof: more calls on Monday.

Living in an impatient culture where, once we have made a decision, we want action now – like making a major purchase or looking for a new job – and health care is the same. The definition of an emergency is subjective.

Bob Geldof wrote the song with this title using the quoted and extreme reason given by an American child who had sprayed her class with an automatic weapon one Monday in January 1979. It is the day of frustration and relief, planning and sorting.

But, as it is predictable, it should be manageable too.

Whether we are dealing with the GP surgery, the outpatient clinic of the hospital or the routine baby-weighing sessions run by health visitors, many of the principles below apply. Involved in our dysfunctional appointment system is a group consisting of all ranks of clinicians (doctors and nurses), the manager and the support staff. And we have all been at meetings to discuss the problem.

Table 11.1 was developed using the 'yes, but' school of management.

This frivolous exercise is merely to show that no change occurs in isolation and that an improvement in one part of the system is likely to show up adversely elsewhere. Yet the answer GPs and other doctors give to many issues – more resources please – is not politically realistic and is not necessarily the only step forward either.

Frustration builds in the meeting and the doctor wishes to settle on a solution, but, as in previous chapters, we are discussing the limits of clinical responsibility. We find that this manager–doctor line is drawn in different places by different practices, perhaps reflecting the personalities involved.

A weak manager might capitulate to the GP and become an administrator, doing as he or she is told and accepting a clear hierarchy from senior clinician to him or her. Such managers are common in primary care, feeling overwhelmed by the intellectual weight and status of especially the senior doctors. The GP here tends to go into problem-solving mode and has ideas to patch up issues.

'What do you want to do about the clinic running late, doctor?' 'Tell the patients to be on time.'

Table 11.1: Reasons for failing to solve the appointments problem

Problem (apparently)	Proposed change	Yes, but
Surgery always starts late because clinicians arrive late	Set target of being punctual	The doctors, not being idle, have other things to do – when will they do them?
Patients waiting over half an hour. Some patients arrive very early	Set system to monitor patient flows and bring in extra staff where need is predicted	Clinic is often slow because the patient was late (bus timetable?). Extra staff not available. Patient flows uneven
The end of the clinic is always over an hour late. The last patient waits a long time	Make appointment times longer	Some patients need only a short appointment. Cannot be sure in advance which ones
Cannot get through on the phone, especially Mondays	Ask patients to phone on other days	They won't, because they discussed the problem with family at the weekend
Missed appointments	Strict policies, letters sent to patients, sanctions	The GP uses the time to catch up, so becomes stressed if there are no 'did not attends' during the clinic
Unclear follow-up instructions for staff	Get the GP to write them down	GP can't find the form, or can't do this on the computer
Telephone calls to the doctor keep interrupting the GP	Ban them; stop them at reception	The calls are important and it takes 15 minutes to sort out later when three would have solved it earlier
Emergencies disrupt the clinic	Alter the emergencies rota so someone else handles the emergency calls	That means the same people end up doing all Monday emergency calls
Extra patients booked at the last minute	Cater for them with scheduled slots	Reception staff fill them as 'routines' because they like to be kind
No coffee; staff have insufficient time	Coffee machine (20p plastic cups)	Rebellion

One form of unconfident GP, unenthusiastic about solving the problem, might elect to duck his or her role in conversing with management altogether. These GPs potter in, see their allotted patients and go off. They might complain privately but not make a public fuss about problems; they might well be rather legalistic and stick very much to some contract or other. They might or might not attend the discussion, but not contribute. This means managers are in danger of setting unrealistic targets and priorities for the want of sound advice, and fail to use resources ideally.

Another doctor despairs of the chaos and tries hectoring or even bullying. Then the performance of everyone involved inevitably drops off and, although the manager knows he or she has to stick around, clinical colleagues disappear as fast as they can.

Problems multiply as the manager tries to run the system for 52 weeks with 44 weeks of staff presence, spending more time on crisis-aversion this week than thinking about next month. So someone, usually the manager, suggests another team meeting to make some decisions.

Trust and teams

How quaint that the reforms of the last 15 years have abandoned hospitals and authorities and developed trusts. Such a positive word, hopeful and simple, designed to help us know that they are there to take the weight off our shoulders and not worry.* Perhaps we should look at trust rather than trusts and see why this is a problem.

After all are we doctors not exhorted to work in and with teams now, with multiple professions co-operating to formulate the best plan for the patient? Team-working is a must-have jargon term for any ambitious practice trumpeting its successes (and fishing for more money). But what is a team?

They need a common goal and that in itself might not be easy to identify and agree on. We have discussed the way that in a consultation patients are not always able to put their cards on the table and express their concerns, and indeed the one with the concerns and who needs reassurance or explanations might not even be in the room. Individuals in a team are prone to the same problem: their idea of the team goals might be hard to express. There might be all sorts of barriers to openness:

- the atmosphere of the discussion might be intimidating

- the team might have an idealist who is prone to whipping up enthusiasm until the team sets an absurd goal. Others don't wish to be the killjoy who reins in the plans

- a team member might feel that he or she has a personal agenda, like picking the kids up from school, which conflicts with the team's ambitions, and doesn't want to express it for fear of seeming like a wimp

- there might be genuine clinical differences of opinion. Setting a goal to run a particular aspect of the service to, say, improve cholesterol levels in hypertensives might convince some more than others of its cost-effectiveness.

---

* Some employees of trusts might feel that in this regard they do not succeed but I could not possibly comment.

The GP needs to feel a responsibility, however, to decide on his or her personal priorities and the extent that they are negotiable. It might be that picking the kids up is not negotiable and anything the team does which threatens that will have to be vetoed. If the veto is to be used, then great consideration must go into that: decide if it is reasonable and discuss it with the team leader/chair. The test of reasonableness is going to include contractual obligations – if one has a job or agreement that clearly states 9–5 and now it is impossible for you to work after 3.30 then something has to go and it might be you, or some income. But the open approach of coming clean is far better than bitterly submitting to team will, when the team has not understood the issues. It is not displaying vulnerability to air personal goals and needs. The public veto, however, is a last resort rather than a first one.

Within functioning medical teams there is a consensus about where they want to be in a given timescale (this is called the Development Plan), which works if some time was set aside to meet as a group. This should be well chaired, ensuring everyone has a chance to take a step back and look at the practice's aims. Everyone should keep to discussing first the desired outcomes rather than the processes (which need looking at later). The group needs to have a few simple ideas, not a long complicated list after the exercise. And it needs to be sensitive to cues dropped in by the team members as asides or jokes that actually indicate strong contrary feelings about an issue. Decisions then become deliverable.

One way of moving the discussion on is to allow what seems at first to be completely unrealistic ideas to be brought in. If a team is aware that access is a problem, a discussion might quickly wander off into weekend or evening working and all those who feel their long days are quite long enough immediately reach for the protest banners. But exploring the problem more might lead to radical solutions: some workers might like weekends if they had weekdays off (helps with the school pick-up problem); taking on weekend staff might be justified by the increased income; or different staff doing different roles and so on. However, it might not, and at worst the problem might be left unsolved. The act of airing it will have helped the team and at least removed a misperceived threat of compulsory weekend working or whatever. The decisive doctor is prepared to speak out.

Group rules, disruption and competitive perfectionism

The underlying competitiveness of doctors is like a market force: potentially we all gain somewhat but it certainly needs regulating, and many situations are better off without it. A really strong team could discuss this, but it all gets a bit close to personality issues and counselling, and all that alarming and boggy area, for many GPs. More reasonably is to agree some Group Rules and anyone who has run a small group knows the value of these. The first rule is that all the other rules are agreed by the group – not imposed – and written down, and not really thereafter negotiable. It is like a mini-constitution.

The aim is to keep the team working together and not let an individual mess it up, yet let all individuals feel respected.

A team would consider headings for group rules such as:

- punctuality, meeting timings

- dress, respectful language

- equality

- relevance

- commitment.

And of course anything else.

Many of these are aimed at sorting out the petty irritations of life like persistent lateness or overbearing domination of meetings; it gives the group authority to impose its will where needed, usually through the chair. If there weren't group rules then goals would be missed because everyone is being too courteous and not saying anything to the member who seems to be the problem.

Competitive perfectionism is a term that has been used to describe a particular behaviour of physicians in their communications with each other.[2] If the doctors are in the same team but have different goals, which might be in conflict with each other, then one response is a display of competitive perfectionism. This is otherwise known as point-scoring. The remarks of the player are aimed at both demonstrating superior wisdom to the others and putting down one or more colleagues – indirectly, but that is what it feels like.

It is linked to perceived autonomy. When a GP wants to just get on with the job and not be harassed by the demands of other people and their worries, he or she is asking to be left alone. He or she seeks a kind of uncritical autonomy, a quiet life perhaps. When this is threatened as it must be in any modern, accountable system, GPs rush to justify themselves and prove their worth. Competitive perfectionism is a sign of anxiety. Nervous doctors struggle to trust colleagues to do things in the way they wish and tend to behave as if their method is the only way of doing things. It is possible they have some evidence to back this up but the colleagues are insufficiently well read to be able to argue against it. It is also sometimes a sign of intellectual stasis: I do this because I have always done this. Such GPs are asking to be trusted – which is fine – but not measured and audited – which is not acceptable.

Where a team member is a persistent problem then the team has to discuss it. There will be a weighing up of the options of confrontation, change, break-up or acceptance. The latter course, if chosen, must be a positive choice even if it emerges as the least bad option rather than the best. It is not a good idea to keep revisiting the same issue unless there is something new to discuss.

Who is in the team anyway? And who's in charge around here?

This book is aimed at primary care clinicians, and in discussing teams it is those teams that involve more than one clinician. Some small general practices have only one doctor and if they have no nurse with any autonomy then perhaps they are a rare example of truly working singly. Our single-handed GP likes the control he or she believes is gained, and has a hierarchical structure of support in doing the work, which leads to the outcomes the GP alone sets. However, even these GPs are not wholly isolated, much as they would wish it. Their income is set by parameters and goals with which they might not agree, and their work is supervised by outside managers from the Primary Care Organisation (PCO). Such GPs are an endangered species, but at their best have great diversity and flexibility (and, at their worst, quite the reverse).

The style of the dictatorial doctor-boss is not readily adopted in any other situations: we have to talk to each other. The majority of us have to get on with a batch of fellow GPs whom we didn't appoint and whom at first we don't know.

By working a bit in other environments (outpatients, out-of-hours centres, commissioning and politics) many GPs will be in more than one team. They have to be aware of the benefits of this (careful implantation of ideas might result in progress, rather like putting tomato genes in genetically modified wheat) and the drawbacks (conflicts of interest when the wheat field overruns the tomato patch). It might be they have to have one team that commands their main loyalty but all the teams need to understand this.

Of course the leader of the group is by convention the oldest member in primary care. In contrast many hospital directorates will have a volunteer director from amongst the consultants. Neither is necessarily by appointment, competition or merit but almost certainly he or she will be a doctor. One can argue the merits of this, and there is a considerable literature about leadership in medicine. Certain courses are offered; qualifications are obtainable. Yet the confident, successful medical leader often has particular personality it seems, gaining these skills through observation more than tuition, and not necessarily simply by getting older.

The multi-disciplinary team

How can it not be a good idea for patients if varied groups of clinicians discuss cases and formulate a list of actions? The multi-disciplinary team (MDT) is an established feature of the clinical landscape now, though one wonders if some groupings need some weeding. GPs often try to set up a regular meeting with all the practice-attached community and employed clinical staff to discuss cases, and are occasionally involved in MDTs about difficult mental health or paediatric problems.

The objective of the range of clinicians might be an essential method of coming to the best clinical options for the patient. In the ideal meeting there are present all the clinical decision makers about care with the exception of the patient (ahem!), and all those involved know the patient or case or have an academic expertise that can contribute. There is a trade-off in efficiency, however. Problems arise such as:

- rarely will all the team be there
- the team meeting will be scheduled, and regular, but that means delays in decisions until the meeting happens

- the meeting might well be dominated by a particular doctor

- the meeting is used more for updating everyone than for decision making, and this could be done in writing

- any large team meeting is hugely expensive in terms of patient contact time taken out of the week. For any team members who are part-time this effect is much greater: the half-timer could lose 10 per cent of his or her week to meetings but the full-timer only half that

- team decisions can be very conservative and minimal. An unconfident team member driven by risk-aversion will tend to have a strong influence on the case being discussed.

But there are other benefits to holding the meeting even if the patient gain might not be quite as good or clear or obvious as advertised. The individual team members, by the very act of meeting, gain mutual support and understanding of the roles of the other team members. This will pay dividends in the one-to-one conversations held about patients in the intervals between meetings. It is much more than putting faces to telephone voices; the meeting generates an understanding of people's capabilities. This is above and beyond what the team member has been taught: what the other member's profession can or cannot do, and is more personal. One might have an idea what the midwife or community psychiatric nurse (CPN) does, but what is really valuable is knowing what this midwife and that CPN do or are prepared to do. This is education that cannot be achieved any other way and the GP will put some effort into this, even if some of his or her expensive time in the meeting is also spent doodling.

Like any other meeting, therefore, the MDT needs periodically to be reflective.

Does the meeting achieve anything?

Let us move back to the committee, generally the partners' meeting, tackling the appointment problems. The meeting will have an agenda, but only loosely titled, and it might have a discussion paper of varying quality prepared by the manager. The fascinating phase of the proposed change is where the power now lies: can our manager get the appointment system to work better through firm control and rules, with targets like the present 48 hour access and half-hour waits dominating the horizon? Or does the doctor need to defend his or her corner with either an attempt to micro-manage the situation ('Can't Doris the cleaner have her coffee break later so she can get the staff drinks organised?') or a stressed shouting match about being expected to run a teaching session at 8.30 a.m. and yet be in surgery by 9.00 a.m., when it takes ten minutes to boot up the computer and another ten to sign the 'urgent' scripts left helpfully on the desk? The meeting here is short of its goal, and this is partly because the manager's goal is different from the doctor's, and each is inclined to suspect, or even insinuate, that the other is somehow less valuable. In primary care the conflict might be unspoken and be more between the doctor-manager, who has the appointment performance goal, and the doctor-worker, who has a different priority, than the traditional practice manager versus doctor. But the tension is there.

So what might be the goal of a well-organised appointment system? One could put this at a number of levels. It ensures that:

- the surgery runs in a timely, smooth manner

- the patient understands the system

- the patient pathway through the surgery is suitable and reasonably short

- the doctors and nurses are able to do everything they can and need to for the patients

- the patients who are attending really need to be there

- problems that arise can be handled properly by the appropriate person

- there is feedback and monitoring. And the senior management is approachable about intractable issues.

This is a big management agenda. For the inexperienced GP to deal with this is going to be like the medical student caring for the diabetic – he or she knows something about it, is aware of some of the complexities, but might lack the skill and judgement to deliver it well. Yet the experienced GP is jaded by past failures, each new ideas confounded by different factors. This does not stop our fresh doctor from trying, of course, and the less assertive manager lets them, but the confident GP, despite there being so much at stake, might consider trusting the manager to manage.

The manager is being asked to ensure that this is what happens preferably within a budget and with minimal risks. Conflict between goals cannot be avoided, merely understood and prioritised. For instance the goal of 'doing everything they can for the patients' might involve too much time used and conflict with 'timely, smooth manner'. The 'short patient pathway' might conflict with the phlebotomists' schedules and the attempt to 'only see patients who need seeing' involves vetting and questions of who does it and when it can be done. The tension within the team of GPs and manager will blow up when the line of responsibility is not clear. The duty of the decisive GP is to clarify the principles rather than devise detailed solutions.

The dynamics of the meeting

Doctors are invited to meetings as a way of sorting issues out all the time. Frequently this is at the PCT or trust and what follows is perhaps more relevant to those meetings than in-house ones. Attending at least some meetings is part of the GP role, and not one to be completely resented, but a critical view of these matters is wise (see Table 11.2).

Table 11.2: The good and the bad meeting

The bad meeting	The good meeting
Meets because they met last month and they all enjoyed it	Meets when needed, which might be monthly or might not
Agenda set and dominated by one person	Anyone involved can influence the agenda and knows how to
Free-ranging discussion involves much gossip and speculation	Stays relevant (or keeps the gossip to the coffee break)
Chair has not understood the point of the meeting. Information needed by group therefore not thought about in advance and not available	Has an authoritative but inclusive chairman
Has a lot of people present	Has the minimum number present and knows if more than about six, then decisions will be minimal
Very few of whom contribute	Everyone there knows what they are there for and so contributes when it is helpful to the meeting goal
Tries to be inclusive and makes the decision that is least offensive by instinct to everyone – the lowest common denominator	Can be imaginative, can be courageous
Forgets the patient	Thinks whether it will help Mrs Smith
Paperwork circulated at the meeting	Paperwork is short, well written and presented a week beforehand. Members are expected to have read it
Chair uses meeting to rubber-stamp his or her decisions	Chair is essentially neutral, but is empowered to be decisive outside of the meeting if necessary and accountable
Meets in personal time, e.g. breakfast, lunch, evenings	Uses a minimal amount of paid time
Minutes circulated just before next meeting	Meeting members have action points after meeting and do some work between meetings

Clearly if one analyses meetings like this, then the problems they have can be looked at constructively.

The time that a meeting is scheduled is interesting and gives an indication of the thinking behind the event. Why do doctors agree to early morning or evening business-type meetings? Is it because they want to show everyone how hard they work? More status issues perhaps, like an American power-breakfast to demonstrate to the other people present and their colleagues (who will surely know of the meeting) that every waking hour is filled with work and the thought of work? Or is it to demonstrate that the care of patients is too important to be interrupted to discuss, well, the care of patients?

Perhaps doctors like to use meeting times as a weapon, to test the enthusiasm of the proposer of the meeting to carry it through?

Perhaps managers play the same game, thinking that a management meeting is an extra to the day, which would be better spent entirely on real management.

Whatever the history and meaning behind when a meeting is held, the players of the game need to understand the rules. If a participant is reluctant, and making a point by agreeing only if the meeting is inconvenient to others, then his or her membership of the group has to be looked at. If this is an avoidance tactic by the meeting member – he or she doesn't want the meeting to discuss the location of the new bicycle shed to take place because he or she wants a new central heating system instead – then the chair has to discuss it individually away from the meeting. It might be that a previous decision has to be re-confirmed in order to move on.

Meeting length is related to meeting scheduling, since breakfast and lunch meetings will often have an enforced finish time. After all, there is some real work to be done today too....

Primary care clinicians seem peculiarly prone to a dreaded combination of a weak chair and an evening meeting, after a full day's work. This occurs when the agenda is massive, and when the participants can't think of any other way of making it uninterrupted.

The fear that a meeting might decide something the GP is unhappy about drives his or her attendance, since the first rule of power games in even a small institution is understood to be that

> power goes to those who turn up.

This is poor thinking by doctors. If they feel that the point of a meeting is only to protect their own interests, it is not a management meeting they need to be at but a personnel one, or possibly a Local Medical Committee (LMC) meeting. Their attendance at the meeting in this way can make them look self-absorbed and rather territorial, which might not be the case.

NHS management meetings even at primary care level, and certainly at others, seem not to have learned a lot from our democratic systems, which mercilessly use time to force meeting attendees to make decisions about what is important. Shortage of parliamentary time kills off much proposed legislation – not the simple merits of the idea. MPs passionate about one bit of legislation or another might feel frustrated when schedules squeeze them off the agenda, but it is the safest way of keeping to what matters most. The system will tend to default to no-change and the issue can be resumed if there is enthusiasm for it later. It is open to government manipulation, and subject to party disciplines, but all democracies do this to some degree. Where there is a quorum system then change cannot happen without sufficient interest in it. So perhaps more accurately

> power to change things goes to those who turn up (if enough do so).

For clinicians to trudge along to meetings, then, just to ensure their interests are looked after is illogical; they should just ensure the meeting has a clear set of goals, a defined time to look at them, and therefore no surprises.

Someone else's problem

Regrettably GPs (and even more so, some hospital doctors) on the ground find it too easy to say or imply to patients that

> what I think you need is X but *they* won't pay for it.

We can indulge in some speculation about the doctor from this remark. Almost all these show the clinician up in a poor light.

The following list gives reasons for why this might be so.

1. The clinician is feeling isolated. Is this because of feeling undervalued, that resources tend to go elsewhere? Or that no one asks him or her? Or that he or she doesn't know who to ask? Perhaps the GP here has a learning need. He or she might need to discover something about working in teams. Perhaps the GP does not understand the NHS manager's job and instead of spending two days at a Continuing Personal Development (CPD) conference he or she could use the time to shadow someone. The GP might need to learn to accept corporate decisions, and if he or she has no personal desire to go into management then he or she should support those who do. This is the 'what am I here for?' approach for the doctor.

2. 'They' is undefined and yet implies uncaring managers/government and politicians/bosses rather than any rational, approachable decision-making process. This is weak cynicism at best. To suggest to a patient that the management is not interested in him or her is factually wrong. Doctors must work from the premise that managers have the same values they have: they work for money and the good of the patient. Human nature would also suggest that when a manager is needed to support a clinician, say over a complaint, the clinician who has taken the cynical approach might have his or her fears met.

3. The GP or hospital doctor is not keen to take responsibility for the clinical decision he or she is considering. If a GP feels he or she has to take responsibility for the total health of his or her patient, that the patient is a passive recipient of care, then the burden will prove to be too much. The GP needs to deflect the responsibility to an agreement between him or her and the patient, not to some distant authority. The decision if joint will always be better.

4. The clinician is interested in a new but unproven, or at least not widely accepted, therapy and wants to try it. The NHS can be ponderous about bringing in new therapies and the private sector can appear more attractive in this way. Culturally, British medicine is conservative and sceptical of the belief, prevalent in the private sector of the USA and some of continental Europe, that new means better. So we use old, proven antihypertensives that

we understand well, and we resist – to an extent and for a while – the market penetration of new ones. We do not perhaps have a need, like a car manufacturer or a Harley Street clinic, to appear at the forefront of development and change. Yet, of course, massive amounts of research leading to effective change do occur in the NHS without being perceived by patients. Our GPs are less confined than in, say, an HMO (health maintenance organisation) in the USA, which has tramlines of protocol-driven care, of proven benefit, to ensure efficiency. The doctor who feels that he or she wants to try experimental work in the NHS has ways of doing so – slow, perhaps, but they are there. He or she needs to learn to share these thoughts with the patients. And accept that there are mechanisms through which innovations can become mainstream practice, for instance through NICE.

5. The GP feels any restriction on his or her clinical freedom because of budgetary issues is immoral. Mixing up spending priorities with morality is unworthy. Unglamorous areas of the NHS like learning difficulties services, mental health, dermatology, pathology, even until recently primary care, and so on, are prone to believe that they receive less interest because the papers are not excited by their work. A new technique giving a modicum of relief for a rare form of psoriasis or enuresis gets less publicity than cancer surgery or heart transplants yet quite possibly gives greater health gain. But the management systems for evaluating the new ideas are there, and attempt objectivity more than GPs might acknowledge. Sometimes cost benefits are important. And to isolate one's own field as more morally worthy than another is to misunderstand health care in a democracy.

So should doctors mention treatments that are not (yet) available? Certainly patients are interested in the new and exciting developments in health and it sells a lot of newspapers. But patients are of the same conservative culture as we are, indeed probably more so (we've all met with 'I'm not one for taking tablets') so it is quite fair to burden a patient with the knowledge that there are new ideas out there, that they might or might not be useful, and at the moment the NHS is waiting and seeing. It is a justifiable and acceptable philosophy.

Rationing

The need for rationing is implicit in any healthcare system even if politicians are not able to use such a strong word. The conflict between doctors and managers is often around the use of resources and the effect this has on patient care. Here above all the GPs, even as patient advocates, need to see that the priorities are not theirs to set, on a strategic scale. They might well be able to choose between priorities in their zone: the purchase of one bit of kit instead of another, or the appointment of one type of support staff rather than another. The bigger stuff, from primary care commissioning upwards, is more difficult.

One might yearn for leadership here. The case of Child B was a case where the use of resources was carefully considered and the NHS correctly decided to withhold treatment in a most tragic case.[3]

Child B – Jaymee Bowen

In March 1995 Jaymee was 10, and had acute myeloid leukaemia (AML). She had survived to the age of five with acute lymphoblastic leukaemia (ALL) yet had then developed the AML and was thought to be terminally ill at this point, with a predicted eight weeks to live. Other than palliative care, the only therapy her regular clinicians at Addenbrooke's Hospital, Cambridge, had to offer was a second bone marrow transplant and intensive chemotherapy. They felt strongly that this was not in Jaymee's interests and didn't want to do it, but her father found a clinician on Harley Street, Dr Garvett, who was prepared to carry it out. Jaymee's father took the health authority (HA) to court to get the £75,000 to pay for treatment and won, but on appeal the HA's decision was upheld. Publicity flared up around the case, and Jaymee's therapy was paid for by a benefactor. In the end she had neither a second transplant nor standard intensive chemotherapy but an experimental treatment called donor lymphocyte infusion. Jaymee went into remission and sought further funds for more experimental treatment.

The Chief Executive of Cambridge and Huntingdon HA, Steven Thornton, publicly backed his HA's decision and received a large amount of adverse publicity, vilified for allowing the accountants to dictate treatment decisions. Jaymee, her family forgoing anonymity, herself appeared on TV, angry with the 'managers'.

In the event she lived several months longer than predicted, eventually succumbing to the disease.

The publicity around the treatment decision was emotional and not entirely informative, since the case could so easily be used for substantiating other claims like wastefulness and bureaucracy by those with a different agenda.

The case was not about rationing or money; if £75,000 was needed to save her life then there was and is no question of finding it. The case was an issue of boundaries, of where the NHS draws a line at futile or experimental treatments, where patients in desperation have hopes that appear unrealistic.

Steven Thornton was notably courageous in defending the decision. The clinicians were reasonable, though seemed rather absent from the firing line.

Thornton was taking massive responsibility and the doctors around him must have been very grateful that he was prepared to do so; the decision was corporate, not his alone, but he clearly supported them. Would the average Professional Executive Committee (PEC) chair have stood up to be counted?

Launching a new idea

The GP might well have an exciting new idea for a service development that he or she is keen to see in place. It is vital that GPs understand to whom they should speak about this because there is much confusion.

Approaching the commissioner

Within a Primary Care Organisation (PCO), for instance, a service development will depend on whether anyone is interested in buying it, which from GPs will be usually termed an enhanced service, or might now be part of the Practice-Based Commissioning (PBC) system. There will be a forum for the discussion, but the main changes occur perhaps just once a year as a contract is negotiated with the PCO and so a commissioning decision of any size can be very slow. The primary care team who came up with the plan would need in the first instance to discuss this with the management in the PCO.

Beware the chief executive's gambit

A physiotherapy service believed it had a new way of dealing with respiratory patients that was the best thing ever. A senior manager of some experience discussed it with the physiotherapy service.

Superintendent physiotherapist: 'I have a brilliant idea. It's really important.'

Chief executive: 'Tell me about it.'

'We can do X, Y and Z for these asthmatics. It will save money in the long run. We need to start doing it now. My colleagues are on board and keen. They are already doing it at St Elsewhere's.'

'That sounds good. But how important is it compared with all your other work?'

'It is one of the most important things we would do.'

'Well how about we do it, but you must tell me the least important thing you are doing at the moment.'

'But everything we do is important.'

'Oh. I think that may be a problem.'

There are off-the-peg schemes for many situations that nevertheless need some tailoring. The PCO might well have made the first move too but the management in the primary care team needs to try to lead the decision making to ensure the PCO's ideas fit into the primary care team's overall plans.

Proposers tend to feel that the way to a manager's heart is through the budget, and most new ideas are somehow shown in the early paperwork to save money in the long run somewhere else in the system. They suggest the new drug will prevent operations and admissions, the new procedure will lead to earlier discharge, the new nutrition system will have them recovering in no time, and the new community support will prevent loss of independence and emergency admissions. Always the problem is that the proposer is suggesting that a modest investment in his or her department will lead to savings in someone else's.

The more recent proposals for community matrons have this flavour as a result of the research done in the USA, although this has been much criticised. GPs, however, are not averse to the tactic – they like to have, say, better access to ultrasound because it would 'save referrals and the hospital radiology unit' but instead the tendency in practice will be to lower the threshold for having a scan done because it is now so convenient.

So, regrettably, the reality is that such savings often fail to materialise. The department that benefits from better patient care elsewhere will have other good ways of spending its money and will be able to demonstrate just how vital its service is.

But when asked to identify savings in his or her own areas, as above, the proposer rather dries up.

Actually the manager might just be interested in the fact that the new idea improves patient care: there are expanding budgets, there are ways. It's a management problem.

The solution looking for a problem

There is a particular hazard in an era of change that a doctor becomes enthusiastic about a computer system, a piece of equipment or a technique without being entirely clear what the problem is that needs solving. We then become advocates for an improvement of some sort that is unproven. If the meeting at which this is discussed also suffers from some of the faults discussed above, then a poor decision might be made and, obviously, the management is blamed. There is a danger of adopting a position of uncritical certainty about a solution, when uncertainty is more objectively justifiable.

The parallel as usual is with primary care consulting. The patient approaches us immediately, as he or she sits, asking for a sick note, or antibiotics, or physiotherapy as a solution to his or her problem before the issue has been fully explored. The problem from the patient's perspective is already clear and encapsulated in a single phrase 'for my sore throat' or 'to help my arthritis'. The confident GP's approach is to start at the beginning, however, and listen carefully before considering the options for a solution. The GP has to hear the patient's diagnostic ideas but has a duty to make his or her own mind up.

In a meeting considering an innovation, at the risk of being accused of excessive caution, a careful history is well worth taking.

Conclusions

The idea of team-working is appealing to management consultants and politicians but the NHS is a mess of teams, ill defined and unclear in their goals. When it works it improves efficiency, possibly for indirect reasons such as getting to know other professionals rather than because of better clinical decision making. The complexity of the dynamics in a meeting has to be understood by the interested, decisive GP. There is a duty to understand rationing and even support it. With whatever systems GPs work they need to be conscious of constraints and be focused on them to the exclusion, if necessary, of other matters (see Appendix 1).

153

References

1. Davies P. The beleaguered consultation *British Journal of General Practice* 2006; **56**: 226–9.

2. Akre V, Falkum E, Hoftredt B, *et al*. The communication atmosphere between physician colleagues: competitive perfection or supportive dialogue? A Norwegian study *Social Science and Medicine* 1997; **44**: 519–26.

3. Entwistle VA, Watt IS, Bradbury R, *et al*. Education and debate: media coverage of the Child B case *British Medical Journal* 1996; **312**: 1587–91.

An exercise for the effective team

The theory of constraints

As a visible and dynamic allegory for the NHS, the M25 London orbital motorway has many features to help us understand this great institution.

Obviously it is circular, and therefore has no end.[*] It is immensely important and useful to huge numbers of people who nevertheless loathe it. Everyone wants to use it at the same time. The very existence of the motorway attracts traffic, in much the same way as the development of new services in the NHS tends to create work. This might be an overall benefit in that previously unfulfilled needs are now met, or it might be that people managed quite well until they were told they needed something. The service quickly becomes a right rather than a privilege and when the system clogs up it becomes a major nuisance.

The behaviour of individuals on the road is also instructive. We have all trundled along the motorway at our usual speed, come to the rear of a queue, and stopped. The line edges along, as drivers continually monitor the other lanes for signs of favouritism and weigh up the risks and hassles of darting between lanes, versus a relaxed, live-longer approach. Duly, the traffic speed picks up and rushes off, yet no clear obstruction is apparent. There were no cones, no hard-shoulder wreckage to admire, no blue lights. The heavy traffic just seemed to clog the road for a while before trundling onwards. And another meaningless queue forms a few miles later.

Seen from above the cars are accelerating to 70 and above, only to swiftly decelerate to walking pace and below. The driver naturally tries to make up for lost time spent in the queue by moving up the next stretch as fast as possible. It creates the kind of Mexican wave effect seen in football crowds.

The conditions for this type of road behaviour are when the traffic flows become both thick and fast. Initially everyone is belting along, drivers alert and aware that all the traffic is bunching a bit, but deducing that, if everyone sticks to their speed, distances between cars should remain unchanged. The wave on the motorway starts when one driver, marginally too close to the next, touches his or her brakes probably quite lightly. The red brake lights alarm the car behind, who is

---

[*] And possibly no point.

also injudiciously close, and the driver finds he or she is rapidly gaining on a braking vehicle. The driver touches his or her brakes as a reflex, but a little more strongly because this is a bit alarming. The first car had only decelerated by 3 m.p.h., but the next one drops by 5. Within seconds the line behind slows more and more. As the cars are very close to each other, technically too close even at much slower speeds, the cars further back end up decelerating hard. Frequently the traffic stops completely.

You can model this mathematically. But the M25, or any busy motorway, shows it well. However, improvements to flow arose when speed limits of 30 or 40 m.p.h. were introduced in heavy traffic. At that speed the tendency for Mexican waves and stop-start driving spells lessened. It seems that drivers at the slower speeds could judge the mild decelerations well and did not over-compensate because they knew the safety margin, the stopping distances. They were able to make better decisions about when and how much to brake and accelerate. It works as long as everyone stays within a narrow speed band, and crucially the result is better average speeds; drivers get to their destinations more swiftly. The decision to stop the traffic going at 70 m.p.h. when it was very heavy in those areas seemingly without an obstruction or, for the moment, a Mexican wave, was counter-intuitive, but is now well-proven to be effective. By going more slowly a better average speed is maintained and so traffic actually progresses more quickly, and, almost as a by-product, more safely.

Back to the NHS, and the flows through its system. We are all trying to help patients reach a good outcome, safely and happily, or at least to an optimum state, and we have massively complex systems for doing this. Simplistically, pathways of patients through the NHS can be described, followed and sometimes understood.

We have to bear in mind that what the politicians and our dear leaders seek and pay for is countable and accountable care, and we live in a system that in this sense has a goal that we cannot influence. Accepting the limitations of measuring our work by these demands, why do some units and sections of the NHS and certainly some primary care teams demonstrate better performance than others?

Is it always down to lack of resources and 'we have a difficult case mix'? Certainly it is sometimes, but careful analysis will sometimes show that systems can improve too. This is where is it worth trying to identify the constraints beyond a simplistic 'we don't have enough nurses'.

Patient flows

The original theory of constraints was put forward by a man called Goldblatt in the early 1980s working as a management adviser to US industry. It has accordingly caught on here for the NHS.

Suppose a practice has a large number of diabetics on its list, perhaps from an elderly population or a large South Asian element. The sequence of care for such patients might be:

1. Patient presents either symptomatically or not with possible diabetes

2. The possibility is discussed with the patient face to face or on the phone and (further) tests arranged

3. The patient makes an appointment for blood tests (involving receptionist and phlebotomist time)

4. The patient attends for further blood test, ideally fasting

5. The result is sent to the doctor from the lab, usually electronically, and the doctor views the result, processes it and makes a diagnosis

6. The doctor contacts the patient to convey the diagnosis (uses his or her own time and administration staff time), make arrangements for basic education and testing (the practice nurse), and records and codes this in the record system

7. The patient attends again for this further information and to have a spectrum of initial checks done as per protocol (HbA1c, renal function, assessment of cardiovascular status and risk, fundi, etc). This might be done by the doctor or nurse in the practice (or is sometimes delegated to secondary care)

8. A decision is made whether to refer to secondary care and if so a letter is written and sent. Otherwise go to step 12

9. Wait. Then the patient attends the secondary care unit

10. A letter is received from secondary care in paper form

11. It is read by the doctor and processed into the patient records, these days usually electronically. A whole sub-pathway follows until

12. Treatment is started

13. The patient also has this, his or her first annual check, recorded in their GP records

14. Arrangements are made for home glucose monitoring, usually by the patient supervised by the nurse according to current protocols

15. Patients make repeat medication requests as per practice system

16. In due course the administration system (via audit, recall systems or the repeat prescription system) calls the patient in for review

17. Patients then have a regular appointment with the primary healthcare team, often the practice nurse

18. The patient has to have annual checks including regular blood tests so the administration staff arrange for the tests to be done prior to the annual check

19. Patient attends for the blood tests

20. Results sent to the practice and seen electronically by the doctor

21. Patient attends for the result and for the annual check

22. Sequence resumes or continues, probably at point 15

23. In parallel with this system are regular eye tests and other secondary care departments when involved, e.g. vascular surgeons, renal physicians.

If each section took a similar length of time, and had similar resources, then the system would work wonderfully. It would function smoothly and quickly, if not at full speed because this is real life and there would be minor hiccups here and there.

Unfortunately there are numerous more major hiccups that would confound a smooth pathway for our diabetic patients here. The patient might not accept the diagnosis, not understand the doctor's language, not be able to come to appointments convenient to the primary care team, or not want to come. He or she might forget one or other blood test or turn up on the wrong day. The medication regime for most such patients is very complex and so there is much scope for error and problems developing from that. The desired outcome – good diabetic control and so reduced complications – is best achieved through well-organised care, but the sequence is fraught with opportunity for problems. Add to this a pressure of volume of cases to be seen and decisions made, and the diabetic clinic becomes a familiar bedlam.

The clinic response is to play safe and touch the brake: the patient is brought back a little early, because we are worried we have not sorted out the issue. Yet during the clinic is a tendency to accelerate through the later patients, perhaps because the clinician (GP, nurse, whoever) is tired and no longer in listening mode but becoming mechanical. Something alarming is spotted, though, and the brake is touched again. But the flow that concerns us is not within the clinic but really the annual flow of achieving a certain volume of care for this group of people each year, not just what happens on a bad day. Patients end up spilling into non-diabetic appointments, time is used elsewhere in the practice, or some checks and tests are not done at all. When the system is overloaded the progress through the system of all patients is slowed up – advice is not given, treatments not sorted and problems not identified with data until the audit shows gaps – so work has to be repeated. The result is a poor system that uses resources from elsewhere to keep functioning or fails a number of patients.

The constraint in the system needs identifying. It might be the GP or the nurse's time and energy, or one or other of the administrative processes. If the constraint is, say, phlebotomy appointment times then improving them should improve the speed at which the whole pathway works. But the constraint might be the patients' own education level, or their willingness to engage with the offered care, even if it is ideal on paper. If that is the problem then increasing the medical resource – the availability of the GP – will not help, because that is not the constraint.

The system as described is seen by providers like us as a patient-centred model but actually expects more from a certain cohort of patients than they can do – how to reach the nursing home patients, the ones who don't speak English or a language of the various team members, the alcoholics, all the 'impossible' patients who cannot plug into the pathway, is a GP headache.

Logically the team should identify the constraint in the pathway that works for the majority of the patients and as a team always focus on that constraint – if it is the nurse's time, which cannot be increased, then at least ensure that his or her time is spent doing the work that only he or she can do – not filling in forms, or doing bloods, or even checking the blood pressures (these are for the healthcare assistant perhaps). The maximum efficiency of the system is then maintained – until an 'impossible' or confounding patient is plugged into the system. Such patients are best served by being outside of the sequence rather than using huge resources within it. They need personally tailored care.

Medical teams do not focus quite so easily though. The ethos of individuality and professional responsibility (rather than corporate) makes us a bit reluctant to become proper team players and, anyway, we all like to be team leader.

But if the theory of constraints holds then the team has to agree what the constraining factor is and focus on it. Ultimately the conversation at the team meeting might be:

159

> **GP:** I need time to catch up on administration matters with the diabetic clinic and so I want to cancel it in a month's time so I can complete the reports to be done.

> **Team:** But the constraint in the system is your availability for annual checks so we'll get behind with those and miss the targets.

> **GP:** I won't be idle you know. The paperwork needs doing some time. I want it done before my holiday.

> **Team:** Can't it be done whilst you are on holiday by others, or taken out of some non-diabetic clinic time?

> **GP:** I can't delegate it all but maybe some could be passed on.

> **Team:** The constraint in the system is the one thing not to constrain further so we'll take on those audit reports....

Perhaps this is too idealised. The doctor probably just wants a break from the bedlam.

How do you see medical knowledge?

Think of our professional knowledge as a box....

Cardiology	Urology	Psychiatry	Surgery	Gynaecology	etc.	etc.			

Do GPs know something of everything (above) and specialists everything about something, plus a bit of everything else (below)?

Cardiology	Urology	Psychiatry	Surgery	Gynaecology	etc.	etc.			

Or is there a body of knowledge of primary care alone, covering some areas that no secondary care specialist does?

Cardiology	Urology	Psychiatry	Surgery	Gynaecology	etc.	etc.	Primary care	Primary care	Primary care

There is a large area of clinical medicine that is exclusive to primary care, encompassing complex conditions and needing special expertise just as secondary care clinicians provide in their field. *Remember – you are a specialist.*

Index